HEALTH POLICIES, HEALTH POLITICS

DANIEL M. FOX

Health Policies
Health Politics

THE BRITISH AND
AMERICAN EXPERIENCE
1911-1965

PRINCETON UNIVERSITY PRESS
PRINCETON, NEW JERSEY

Copyright © 1986 by Princeton University Press

Published by Princeton University Press, 41 William Street,
Princeton, New Jersey 08540
In the United Kingdom: Princeton University Press, Guildford, Surrey

All Rights Reserved

Library of Congress Cataloging in Publication Data will be
found on the last printed page of this book

ISBN 0-691-04733-2

This book has been composed in Linotron Palatino

Clothbound editions of Princeton University Press books
are printed on acid-free paper, and binding materials are
chosen for strength and durability

Printed in the United States of America by Princeton University Press
Princeton, New Jersey

CONTENTS

ACKNOWLEDGMENTS

I AM GRATEFUL to many historians and political scientists, whose work I cite in the notes and in the bibliographic essay. Several colleagues were particularly generous throughout this project. John Burnham and Rudolf Klein made many important suggestions. Brian Abel-Smith and Charles Webster helped me to understand British sources and were, along with Lawrence D. Brown and Theodore R. Marmor in the United States, sharp critics of my statements about policy and politics. Barbara Gutman Rosenkrantz corrected a number of errors and made an important contribution to the organization of the book. David P. Willis commissioned some of the early research, commented on early drafts of the manuscript, and sustained my confidence that I had something new to say.

I thank many archivists and librarians in Britain and the United States. I am particularly grateful to the staffs of the library of the Wellcome Institute for the History of Medicine and of the Health Sciences Library at Stony Brook.

Other people and organizations also contributed to this book. Work on this book was financed by a grant from the Commonwealth Fund Book Program and by a sabbatical leave from the State University of New York at Stony Brook. For more than a decade, J. Howard Oaks and Marvin Kuschner have understood my desire to combine research with administration and teaching. The staff of the Office of the Vice President for Health Sciences at Stony Brook typed many drafts of this book and of the papers that preceded it. Gail Ullman of the Princeton University Press was a liberating editor.

INTRODUCTION

MANY of the vexing problems of health affairs in Britain and the United States in the 1980s are the unanticipated consequences of a policy, more precisely, a set of policies and ideals that, for most of this century, seemed self-evidently the best way to advance science and improve the health of the public. I call this policy hierarchical regionalism, by which I mean a particular logic of organization based upon a theory of how medical knowledge is discovered and disseminated.

I use the phrase hierarchical regionalism to summarize three assumptions that became the basis of health policy in Britain, the United States and, I believe, most industrial countries in the twentieth century. These assumptions are: 1) The causes of cures for most diseases are usually discovered in the laboratories of teaching hospitals and medical schools. 2) These discoveries are then disseminated down hierarchies of investigators, institutions, and practitioners that serve particular geographic areas. 3) Health policy should stimulate the creation of hierarchies in regions that lack them and make existing ones operate more efficiently.

This book differs from most accounts of the history of health policy in Britain and the United States in the twentieth century. Most of the accounts describe how each country adopted or resisted policies that distributed the results of the progress of medicine more equitably and efficiently. According to these authors, the goals of proper health policy have been obvious since just after the beginning of this century. Policy should encourage people to seek medical care by providing an adequate and efficiently organized supply of services—doctors,[1] other health workers, and hospitals—and removing or reducing the burden on individuals to pay for them. Most histories of health policy in Britain and the United States describe progress toward these goals. Studies of policy in Britain have emphasized the immediate and remote origins of the National Health Service.[2] Most American students have assumed that their

---

[1] Because the British use the word "physician" to refer only to specialists in internal medicine, I call all members of the medical profession doctors. I apologize to American readers who resent the implication that people who practice medicine have a monopoly on the word "doctor."

[2] Daniel M. Fox, "The National Health Service and the Second World War: The

central task is to explain the failure to achieve compulsory national health insurance.[3]

I write the history of health policy from a different point of view. I try to remain neutral about the worth of particular policies and of the people who advocated or attacked them. In the language of historiography, I am a critic of historicism—of the belief that there is a purpose in history, that events in the past unfold toward the present, and that history teaches. Instead, I try to describe and explain why particular policies were adopted in America and Britain.

Unlike many other historians of health policy, I do not believe that the progress of medicine has made particular policies inevitable or desirable. Instead, I regard as historical data assertions that the progress of medicine creates imperatives for policy. My relativism may disturb some readers, particularly those who are unfamiliar with current work in the history of medicine. In my view, and that of historians whose views I share, medicine changes and advances technologically; but it does not progress. Neither medicine nor the human condition progresses—changes for the best—over time. The purpose, content, and social valuation of medicine are, I believe, in constant flux.

In this book, I describe the effects on health policy of assuming that medicine has progressed and will continue to do so. About a century ago, many people in America and Britain began to believe that, for the first time in history, scientists were discovering wholly new kinds of truths about nature that would, eventually, make it possible for doctors to reduce the suffering and death caused by the most threatening diseases. This sense of discontinuity with the past stimulated new ideas about what health policy ought to do and how it should be done. By the 1920s, health and medical care policy had become synonymous for most people. For the next half-century, health policy was usually made on the assumption that increasing the supply of medical services and helping people to pay for them was the best way to reduce morbidity and mortality and to help individuals lead more satisfying lives. The priority for public health policy in each nation changed from regulating or improving the environment to providing direct services to individuals. Doctors' de-

Elaboration of Consensus," in Harold L. Smith, ed., *War and Social Change: British Society in the Second World War* (Manchester: Manchester University Press, forthcoming).

[3] Daniel M. Fox, "The Decline of Historicism: The Case of Compulsory Health Insurance in the United States," *Bulletin of the History of Medicine*, Winter 1983, 57: 596-609.

cisions about what to order for their patients distributed most of the resources allocated by health policy. Moreover, priority within health policy was accorded to the services provided by specialized doctors in hospitals.

Although I emphasize similarities throughout this book, I am very much aware of the differences between the health policies of the United States and of Great Britain. I stress similarities in order to make clear my major themes: that beliefs drove policy; that beliefs about the implications of medical science for policy transcended national boundaries; and that, as a result of common beliefs, the fundamental organizing principles of health services in the two countries were similar. Policy is what happened when beliefs were, to risk a metaphor, refracted by what, along with other students of history and politics, I call the political culture of particular countries.[4] I have tried to be sensitive to the differences in the political cultures of America and Britain and to how these differences influenced such fundamental issues of health policy as equity, rationing, and the importance accorded to different levels of care.

I have described elsewhere how my experience as both an historian and a public official converged to make me skeptical about the historicist account of the history of health policy.[5] I came gradually and often reluctantly to the interpretations of events I present here.

[4] For an account of the history and definitions of the concept of political culture, see Gabriel L. Almond, "The Intellectual History of the Civic Culture Concept," in G. A. Almond and S. Verga, eds., *The Civic Culture Revisited* (Boston: Little, Brown, 1980), 26ff. With Almond, I define political culture to include structure and style as well as what Talcott Parsons called "psychological orientations."

[5] Daniel M. Fox, "History and Health Policy: An Autobiographical Note on the Decline of Historicism," *Journal of Social History*, March 1985, 18: 349-364.

HEALTH POLICIES, HEALTH POLITICS

I

Health Policy and the Perception of Medical Progress: 1910-1918

IN THE EARLY TWENTIETH CENTURY, many people in both Britain and the United States believed that health policy should be reformulated. Enormous changes were occurring in medicine. For the first time, people of all social classes expected to be hospitalized for serious illnesses. New instruments and techniques made diagnosis more precise. Scientific advances and the publicity accorded them in the press had stimulated optimism that new therapies would soon be discovered. In both countries, more stringent requirements for medical education and entry into the profession combined with the increase in hospital practice had stimulated the emergence of new medical elites. The authority of the members of these elites was grounded to an increasing extent in their knowledge and the prowess imputed to them by colleagues, patients, and by the mass media. Social class still mattered in medicine, but not as much as it had earlier, and considerably less in America than in Britain. Although relationships between the new medical elite and general practitioners were often tense, doctors were, in general, united by a sense of professional solidarity and by a shared commitment to the application of science to medicine.[1]

Politics and society in Britain and the United States were, however, profoundly dissimilar. Britain was a more cohesive society, though with considerable diversity: there are important differences, for instance, among England, Scotland and Wales that are beyond the scope of this book. Nevertheless, debates about policy in Britain occurred among people who, despite frequent disagreements, had a great deal in common. Centralization—of policy and politics, of the allocation of prestige, of the media of communication, of the organizations that represented political and professional interests—made disagreements easier to resolve in Britain than in the United States. Habits of deference restrained the antagonism of

[1] The generalizations in this paragraph and those that follow are based on a rich secondary literature and my own reading of primary sources, which I describe in the "Note on Sources."

3

classes. Moreover, an aristocratic tradition of paternalistic responsibility to alleviate suffering often led to policies that were similar to those derived from socialist theory. The United States, in contrast, was characterized by a more fragmented polity, a fluid class structure, and a narrower range of ideological debate.

Despite these differences, the primary issue for health policy in both nations by 1918 became how to organize and finance medical services. In Britain, every sector of the medical profession and major figures in government, social reform, and voluntary associations were gradually drawn into discussions about organizing and paying for services. In the United States, a coterie of reformers in medicine and philanthropy promoted reorganization while the major associations within the medical profession grew increasingly resistant to it.

Just a decade earlier, organizing and financing medical care was still a subordinate issue in debates about priorities for social policy. Legislators, officials, and leaders of voluntary associations concerned with social problems accorded priority to improving wages and working conditions, preventing or alleviating unemployment, and ameliorating long-term poverty through pensions, education, and improved nutrition.

However, concern about poor health and optimism about medical intervention to remedy it gradually influenced thought and action about social policy after the turn of the century. Social investigators in both nations claimed that illness was a significant cause of poverty. Theorists of human capital and industrialists impressed by new ideas of scientific management argued that healthier workers were more productive. Philanthropists, journalists, and officials were dismayed by the large number of sick children and of adult males disqualified for military service because of poor health. This concern about the health of the working class united imperialists and pacifists, advocates of social insurance and of charity, eugenicists and environmentalists, as well as free enterprisers and socialists. In the United States, the euphemism for improving the health and productivity of the lower classes was "national vitality"; in Britain, it was "efficiency."

In the second decade of the century, compulsory or government health insurance became a public issue in both nations. Within a few years, however, the nature of the problem prominent people in each country wanted to solve with health insurance underwent a profound change. When compulsory health insurance was first proposed, its advocates linked it with social policy to alleviate and prevent poverty. In each nation, however, policy for medical care was gradually separated from general social policy.

By the end of the First World War, the purpose of compulsory health insurance was subtly but decisively redefined. A policy to avoid destitution was transformed into a policy to expand access to desirable services in order to alleviate disease. The organization, financing, and substance of medical services became the central concern of officials and social reformers who were concerned with policy for health.

This redefinition of the problem to be addressed by compulsory health insurance created a major discontinuity in the history of social policy. Social insurance had been instituted in Germany in the late nineteenth century to provide alternatives to socialism. The purpose of social insurance was to reduce the antagonism of the working class toward employers and public officials. In Britain and the United States, similarly, philanthropists and political leaders initially advocated social insurance in order to increase the working class's share of the nation's wealth on terms set by the dominant classes in society. The alleviation of disease, however desirable, was not a central purpose of social policy.

Moreover, the earliest advocates of compulsory health insurance in Britain and the United States described it as an installment on a larger program of social reform. David Lloyd George, chancellor of the exchequer from 1901 to 1914, believed that "at no distant date, [the] state will acknowledge a full responsibility in the matter of provision for sickness, breakdown or unemployment."[2] The American Association for Labor Legislation, which, between 1915 and 1920, promoted a model bill for compulsory health insurance, advocated a program of reform that included improvements in wages, working, and housing conditions and the regulation of collective bargaining.[3]

NATIONAL HEALTH INSURANCE IN BRITAIN

The priority of health policy in Britain changed within a few years from maintaining income to providing services. When, in 1911, Lloyd George introduced national health insurance, his priority

[2] William J. Braithwaite, *Lloyd George's Ambulance Wagon*, ed. by Sir Henry N. Bunbury (London: Methuen and Cox, 1957), 24.
[3] Ronald L. Numbers, *Almost Persuaded* (Baltimore: Johns Hopkins University Press, 1978), *passim.*; Daniel M. Fox, *Economists and Health Care* (New York: Prodist, 1979), 13-14.

was protecting the wages of workers who could not work because they were sick.[4] This policy antagonized influential groups to both his left and his right who worried that workers would be corrupted. To his left, Fabian socialists led by Sidney and Beatrice Webb argued that sick benefits should be paid only to workers who demonstrated willingness to adopt what they called better habits of life.[5] To his right, defenders of a distinction between the deserving and undeserving poor, which had been drawn since Elizabethan times by a succession of laws to regulate the burden of the poor on society and which had been reinforced by conservative Social Darwinism argued, as the author of an unsigned article in the *Times* of London wrote, that "if you offer people . . . relief without any drawback, it is absolutely certain that many will take advantage of it."[6]

Lloyd George modified his program in order to accommodate his opponents' views. Introducing the insurance bill to Parliament in 1911, he conceded that a sick allowance should be paid only to patients who demonstrated deservingness by obeying doctors' orders. Benefits should be conditional on good character rather than an entitlement in all cases of illness.[7] Lloyd George also intended to

[4] On Lloyd George's priorities, "Insurance Scheme," printed "for the use of the Cabinet" in March 30, 1911, and found in the William Braithwaite Papers, British Library of Political and Social Science, Box II.51: "The Bill is intended to effect as wide an insurance as possible of the working class against sickness and breakdown. . . . At the present moment . . . when sickness comes, poverty and distress ensue."

[5] The Fabians' distress at what they considered a misguided emphasis on money was most accessible to contemporaries in Sidney and Beatrice Webb, *The State and the Doctor* (London: Longmans Green, 1910). In their peroration, the Webbs emphasized "personal responsibility" over the "waste and expense of disease" (261). Beatrice Webb told Lloyd George that relief "ought to be conditional on better conduct," according to Norman and Jean Mackenzie, *The First Fabians* (London, Weidenfeld and Nicolson, 1977). The Webbs' antagonism to an income strategy is also documented in A. M. McBriar, *Fabian Socialism and English Politics, 1884-1918* (Cambridge: Cambridge University Press, 1962), and in Kitty Muggeridge and Ruth Adam, *Beatrice Webb: A Life* (London: Secker and Warburg, 1967).

[6] The quote from *The Times* is in Sir Henry Burdett, *The Future of the Hospitals* (London, Spottiswoode and Co., n.d. but probably 1910), 3.

[7] David Lloyd George, *The People's Insurance* (London: Hodder and Stoughton, 1911), 19. This book is a compilation of Lloyd George's contemporary speeches on NHI. *Cf.* David Lloyd George, *The Insurance of the People*, speech at Birmingham, June 10, 1911 (London: Liberal Publication Department, 1911): "Our object, our goal ought to be enough to maintain efficiency of every man, woman and child. . . . The last thing they [the working class] pawn is their pride" (4). But in the same speech—foreshadowing his subsequent ambivalence—he said, "The first thing we do in our Bill is we provide adequate medical treatment for every workman in the kingdom" (8).

expand the scope of health insurance. To organize the program he appointed a junior minister, Charles Masterman, who had written a best-selling book celebrating what he called the progress of the modern campaign against disease.[8] Lloyd George and Masterman planned to mount what they called a "succession of attacks" on specific diseases, beginning with tuberculosis, through health insurance. They chose as administrator of national health insurance a forceful civil servant, Robert Morant, who wanted medical services, not cash, to be the focus of the program. Moreover, Morant wanted the priority of health insurance to be "organizing medical treatment for all wage earners." He hoped that workers would be "enthusiastic consumers" of medical care, even though they "resented compulsory deductions from their wages."[9]

Morant, who was close to the Webbs, was influenced by changing Fabian opinions about health policy. In 1906, Beatrice Webb disparaged what she described as the mere dispensation of physic.[10] By 1910, however, she advocated public and philanthropic policy to extend curative services.[11] Hospitals would increase in number, she assured the British Hospital Association at its first meeting. In 1912, she decided that medical care was part of what she called a war against poverty. The advance of sanitary science, medical and surgical discoveries, and improvements in personal hygiene were, she claimed, the greatest triumph of the nineteenth century.[12] In 1916, she looked forward to a public medical service managing one disease after another.[13] Similarly, by 1918, Sidney Webb, calling for a

[8] C.F.G. Masterman, *The Condition of England* (London: Methuen, 1909), 223-225, 228, 296, 303; Lucy Masterman, *C.F.G. Masterman: A Biography* (London: Nicholson and Watson, 1939), 242, 252, 264. *Cf.* Francis M. Mason, "Charles Masterman and National Health Insurance," *Albion*, Spring 1978, 10: 54-75.

[9] The quotations are from Morant's first memorandum to E. S. Montague, Masterman's successor, in February 1915: in Bernard M. Allen, *Sir Robert Morant: A Great Public Servant* (London: Macmillan and Co., 1934), 288.

[10] Mrs. Sidney Webb, "The Relation of Poor Law Medical Relief to the Public Health Authorities," reprinted from *Public Health*, December 1906, 1-10, in Passfield Papers, London School of Economics, Box VI.65.

[11] Mrs. Sidney Webb, "The Coming of a Unified Medical Service and How It Will Affect the Voluntary Hospital," *The Hospital*, October 29, 1910, 48: 139-145.

[12] Mrs. Sidney Webb, *War Against Poverty: Complete National Provision for Sickness* (London: Independent Labour Party and Fabian Society, 1912) in Fabian Society Papers, Nuffield College, Oxford, E 108/6.

[13] Beatrice Webb, "Lecture on the Professional Organization of Medical Men," 24 January 1916, in B. and S. Webb, *Professional Organization*, vol. I, Passfield Papers, Coll. Misc. 248, London School of Economics. Sidney Webb apparently did not quite agree with Beatrice's opposition to NHI. He assisted Lloyd George to secure trades

threefold increase in hospital beds, asserted that "so long as hospitals are not adequate . . . for all cases requiring them, we cannot get the health of the people improved or premature death postponed."[14]

Leaders of the medical profession also wanted to change the purpose of health insurance from providing cash to purchasing services—from remedying poverty to diagnosing and curing disease. Medical opposition to NHI disappeared quickly as, under it, doctors' incomes rose and their professional autonomy increased because they were freed from what they regarded as the petty restrictions of voluntary group insurance administered by Friendly Societies. Christopher Addison, a doctor who was a member of Parliament and an ally of Lloyd George's, declared in 1914 that he saw no limit to what he called "enlightened cooperation between medicine and the state."[15] With support from the medical profession, Lloyd George and Masterman intended in 1914 to extend insurance to cover specialists' services, but postponed legislation because of the war.

Events during the war accelerated changes in the priorities of health policy. At home, the central government improved and extended the medical services provided by local authorities in order to maintain the productivity of civilian workers despite the absence of half the doctors in military service. More important, the achievements of medicine at the front were widely celebrated. Death rates from contagious diseases and from infections related to wounds were considerably lower than in previous wars, as a result, many experts concluded, of both scientific knowledge and the way services were organized. Emergency surgery in field hospitals had never been so successful. Moreover, military experience increased the number of doctors who had experience of the coordination required to use new machinery for diagnosis and anesthesia. The way services were organized on the battlefield added new words to the vocabulary of civilian medical care: receiving stations, base hospitals, and sectors, for example. As the *Times'* medical correspondent

union and medical support (Lloyd George to S. Webb, March 1, 1911, Passfield Papers, Box II 4.8c e.6). For a different reading of the Webbs and Lloyd George, see Kathleen Woodroofe, "The Royal Commission on the Poor Laws, 1905-09," *International Review of Social History*, 1977, 22: 137-164.

[14] Sidney Webb, *Ministry of Health*. Address delivered . . . at the Annual Conference of the Association of Approved Societies (London: The Association, 1918), 7.

[15] Christopher Addison, *The Health of the People* (London: University of London Press, 1914), 13; *cf.* Kenneth and Jane Morgan, *The Political Career of Christopher, Viscount Addison* (Oxford: Clarendon Press, 1980), 11-12.

said, the war taught both the public and doctors the "value of team-work" and the "need of applied science in medical treatment."[16]

By the end of the war, there was a broad consensus about health policy in Britain. But consensus had been achieved by ignoring the problem of how to measure the extent to which medical care alone was an effective remedy for poverty. The most penetrating analysis of the new health policy was written by William Brend, a barrister who lectured on forensic medicine at Charing Cross Hospital.

Brend was uncertain about whether medical services were an effective remedy for poverty. In 1914 he had asserted that medicine was fighting a winning battle, but warned that it was a mistake to suppose that medical treatment was mainly responsible for preventing sickness or reducing the death rate.[17] Three years later, evaluating National Health Insurance, Brend was still ambivalent about the significance of the progress of applied medical science. On the one hand, surgery had, he said, played a larger part than sewers in the decline of the death rate since the nineteenth century. Moreover, the logic of progress made it inevitable that general practitioners would gradually be replaced by hospital-based specialists. On the other hand, compulsory insurance had failed to improve the health of the working class. Moreover, some of the healthiest people in Britain lived where doctors and hospitals were fewest. Brend could not explain how this mismatch of health status and the location of medical services could exist if access to care were the principal cause of the reduction of sickness and death.[18]

Brend's uncertainties led him to advocate social policy to create more medical services and to raise income and living standards. NHI should be expanded to cover hospital service. The preventive and curative medical services of local authorities should be unified, he wrote. At the same time, he added, the nation needed a broad program of social insurance and housing reform, what the Webbs called the National Minimum.[19]

Most of Brend's contemporaries had no difficulty agreeing with him. They did not find remarkable his inability to determine with precision the contribution of medical progress to social welfare.

[16] Our Medical Correspondent [Robert McNair Wilson], "Health Centers for All: The State and the Doctors," *The Times*, May 26, 1919.

[17] William A. Brend, "The Case for a National Medical Service," *The Nineteenth Century*, June 1914, 1256.

[18] William A. Brend, *Health and the State* (London: Constable and Co., 1917), *passim*. but especially 17, 35, 96, 208.

[19] *Ibid.*, 210-211.

They believed that policy for health should provide more preventive and curative services to individuals. They thought that general social policy should promote a higher standard of living. In the absence of a coherent theory for assigning priority in social policy, it was better to do more rather than less. The Hospital Committee of the British Medical Association, for example, recorded its satisfaction that Brend's book had received favorable comment from the press.[20]

HEALTH INSURANCE IN THE UNITED STATES

The first crusade for state-mandated health insurance in the United States had a different result from the campaign for National Health Insurance in Britain. The coalition supporting the introduction of state laws mandating health insurance became smaller and narrower between 1914 and 1920. When the American Association for Labor Legislation began its campaign for health insurance, it had considerable support among doctors, philanthropists, and some leaders of organized labor. By 1920, a small band of intellectuals, doctors, and laymen, who gave priority to reorganizing medical services, were the most visible advocates of a program that seemed further and further from implementation each year.

The change in emphasis from cash to services among American advocates of compulsory health insurance occurred rapidly and without attracting critical attention. In 1914, a model insurance bill drafted by a committee of the American Association for Labor Legislation accorded priority to what it described as reducing destitution rather than to providing an explicit set of services.[21] Two years later, however, a revised model bill gave priority to remedying the loss of wages due to illness.[22] In 1921, Michael M. Davis, a social scientist who was, like William Brend, a prominent lay expert on health affairs, separated medical services from broad social policy. Sickness was the only cause of poverty that interested Davis. He saw no vicious circle of poverty and illness. In his view, adequate medical service could now relieve and prevent dependency. Amer-

[20] Minutes of Hospitals Committee, British Medical Association. Documents 1917-1918. Meeting of October 9, 1917, vol. 1921. BMA Registry, London.

[21] Numbers, *Almost Persuaded*, 19. For an emphasis similar to mine, see Paul Starr, "The Changing Objectives of National Health Insurance, 1915-1980," in Ronald L. Numbers, ed., *Compulsory Health Insurance: The Continuing American Debate* (Westport: Greenwood Press, 1982).

[22] Numbers, *Almost Persuaded*, 35.

icans, he asserted, should not emulate the British, who temporized about inefficiently organized medical care while they "foolishly" provided cash benefits. Comprehensive insurance in America, Davis maintained, should be deferred until medical care was properly organized.[23]

When the AALL decided in 1914 that compulsory health insurance was the next great step in social legislation, it overestimated its political strength and underestimated the complexity of the issues involved in policy for medical care. The several thousand members of the AALL—most of whom were employed by universities, social settlements and service agencies, or by liberal magazines—were euphoric in 1914. What they called the first step, a campaign to pass laws in the states to compensate workers for job-related injuries, had been a striking success. Irving Fisher, a Yale professor of economics and president of the AALL, had written a stirring *Report on National Vitality* for the Committee of One Hundred, a group of industrial, political and religious leaders appointed by President Theodore Roosevelt.[24] The prestige of social scientists and the civic responsiveness to their sense of mission had never been greater. In 1912, Woodrow Wilson, an academic political scientist, was elected president of the United States. Fisher's views, and those of many of his colleagues in the AALL—John R. Commons, Edward T. Devine, and Henry Seager, for example—were eagerly sought by the press and by public agencies.[25]

The leaders of the AALL misjudged the difference between the politics of national vitality and workmen's compensation and those of compulsory health insurance. The vitality campaign, which linked health to the productivity of workers, occurred at a level of generality that did not create conflict between major interest groups about practical matters. The result of the campaign was a report rather than competition for resources among interest groups. Work-

---

[23] Michael Davis, *Immigrant Health in the Community* (New York: Harper and Bros., 1921), 3, 398. For a very different interpretation of Davis see Ralph E. Pumphrey, "Michael M. Davis and the Development of the Health Care Movement, 1900-1928," *Societas*, Winter 1972, 7: 27-41. Davis's denial of a reciprocal relationship between poverty and disease was unusual. A distinguished contemporary, for example, Homer Folks, believed that "poverty and disease are reciprocally and mutually cause and effect . . . and no one, of whatever profession, can deal effectively with one without taking the other into account at every stage." Quoted in Walter I. Trattner, *Homer Folks, Pioneer in Social Welfare* (New York: Columbia University Press, 1968), 152.

[24] Numbers, *Almost Persuaded, passim.*

[25] Fox, *Economists and Health Care*, 12-14.

men's compensation was a program that had strong support among large employers who were eager to reduce litigation and to increase the productivity of the work force. The new legislation pooled risks within each state and thereby routinized a source of bitter dispute between managers and labor leaders.

Health insurance subsidized by government or employers was, on the other hand, opposed or regarded with skepticism by many individuals and interest groups. Many labor leaders disdained paternalism from either management or government or intellectuals. Some unions provided medical benefits, as they had in Britain before NHI, and labor federations in twenty-one states eventually endorsed mandatory health insurance. But the American Federation of Labor and a majority of its state affiliates opposed it as a distraction from collective bargaining. Employers were uncomfortable about a health insurance program that was also opposed by both the insurance and pharmaceutical industries. Although such leading Progressive politicians as Alfred E. Smith in New York and Hiram Johnson in California endorsed state-mandated health insurance, they were unwilling to take political risks for a program that had little popular support. In public referenda on health insurance, for example, the proponents were routinely defeated.[26] As distaste for state-mandated insurance grew within the medical profession, it was supplemented and reinforced by considerable opposition outside of it.

The American Medical Association and most state medical societies initially supported and then bitterly opposed state-mandated health insurance. This change in the position of organized medicine was, in part, a result of doctors' rising incomes, of conflicts between specialists and generalists, and of the discomfort of many doctors with the suggestion that they should work for salaries or under contracts.[27]

More important, however, the advocates of health insurance made many tactical errors and a crippling strategic mistake. The tactical errors antagonized many doctors. The strategic mistake—insisting that medical practice should be reorganized into hierarchies dominated by specialists—created bitterness against the reformers

---

[26] Numbers, *Almost Persuaded, passim.*, and 91 for referenda. In Britain, in 1910, the Liberal party lost by-elections that turned on the issue of National Health Insurance.

[27] James G. Burrow, *Organized Medicine in the Progressive Era* (Baltimore: Johns Hopkins University Press, 1977), Chapter IX; *cf.* Rosemary Stevens, *American Medicine and the Public Interest* (New Haven: Yale University Press, 1971); *cf.* Paul Starr, *The Social Transformation of American Medicine* (New York: Basic Books, 1982), 243-257.

and their political heirs that persisted for half a century. Organized medicine had mobilized considerable political strength in the states in the first two decades of the century. This power was, after 1920, turned against any innovations in health policy that were associated with mandatory insurance.

The intellectuals who led the AALL made many tactical errors in their campaign for compulsory health insurance. Unlike Britain, for example, where Lloyd George permitted the insurance industry to continue selling death benefits for widows and orphans in order to obtain its support, the American reformers alienated insurance companies by including funeral benefits, a profitable business, in their model bill. Where British politicians created a financial stake in the insurance program for druggists and the manufacturers of pharmaceuticals, the AALL conveyed the impression that hospital pharmacies should dispense all prescriptions.[28]

The British proponents of NHI confronted a different political situation. In the more stratified world of British medicine, NHI was restricted to financing the services of general practitioners. As a result, after 1911 there was hardly any competition between GPs and specialists—consultants in the British usage. The distinction between generalists and specialists in American medicine, especially in large cities, was never as clear as it was in Britain. Where the distinction was clear, moreover, they were usually antagonists.[29] In addition, because Americans had a weaker tradition of voluntary health insurance than the British, they were forced to emphasize innovation rather than to argue from precedent.

Unlike the British promoters of NHI, whose rhetoric was a tool to achieve consensus, American advocates of health insurance, courted antagonism with their words. Irving Fisher, for example, explained in December 1916, a time when American opinion about the war in Europe was becoming increasingly polarized, that Germany had shown the way to compulsory health insurance.[30]

---

[28] See "Note in Sources" for histories of social policy in each country. I do not disagree with Numbers (*Almost Persuaded*, 112), who argues that early support for health insurance was "not confined to a small well-educated elite any more than opposition was restricted to general practitioners." I am persuaded by Numbers's evidence that support was broadly based but I argue that the behavior of the medical intellectual elite helped to convert support into fear of the loss of autonomy and into rage.

[29] Rosemary Stevens, *Medical Practice in Modern England: The Impact of Specialization and State Medicine* (New Haven: Yale University Press, 1966); *cf.* Stevens, *American Medicine*.

[30] Fisher is quoted in Odin Anderson, "Health Insurance in the United States,

Isaac Rubinow, who was the most visible advocate of state-mandated health insurance, caused more damage than Fisher because he insisted that medical practice must be reorganized. For a brief period, Rubinow was both an active member of the AALL and an employee of the American Medical Association. In 1916 alone, he carried his abrasive message to 50,000 people at more than a hundred meetings in eight states.[31] Rubinow, who had degrees in both medicine and political economy, disdained general practitioners because they were, he said, out of harmony with the recent and phenomenal development of scientific medicine. Doctors should only be permitted to practice in an insurance program if they met rigorous standards established by competent authorities. Moreover, except when required by expediency, doctors should not practice alone and patients should not be permitted free choice of doctors.[32] Rubinow also antagonized labor leaders by criticizing workers for regarding insurance from the narrow point of view of immediate financial aid.[33]

American advocates of compulsory insurance were, as Rubinow exemplified, convinced that reorganizing medical care should be the priority of health policy. Health insurance, they insisted, should provide effective services rather than merely replace the wages that were lost during illness. Because the alleviation of disease rather than of poverty became their goal, the organization and substance of services became their dominant concern. The reformers regarded as immoral any compromise that would deprive people of any of the benefits of applied medical science. Money was no substitute for properly organized medical care. To Rubinow, the way most doctors practiced was an anachronism. To Michael Davis, the British and German health insurance programs were retarded at what he called the "stage of individualistic private practice."[34] Richard Cabot, a member of both the social and medical elites of Boston, was more precise. The British and the Germans had failed "to center their medical services around organized groups of physicians—that

1910-1920," *Journal of the History of Medicine and Allied Sciences*, Autumn 1950, 5: 367.

[31] Anderson, "Health Insurance," 369; *cf*. Roy Lubove, *The Struggle for Social Security* (Cambridge: Harvard University Press, 1968), 77, 78.

[32] M. Rubinow, *Standards of Health Insurance* (New York: Henry Holt and Company, 1916), 235, 236-237, 245-246.

[33] I. M. Rubinow, "Health Insurance in Relation to Public Health," *Journal of the American Medical Association*, September 30, 1916, 1014.

[34] Davis, *Immigrant Health*, 398. Cf. Stephen J. Kunitz, "Efficiency and Reform in the Financing and Organization of American Medicine in the Progressive Era," *Bulletin of the History of Medicine*, Winter 1981, 55: 509.

is, around hospitals." A properly organized hierarchy, which was grounded in science and dominated by teaching hospitals was, he said, the prerequisite for an adequate insurance program.[35]

As a result of the tactics and strategies chosen by the crusaders for health insurance, the First World War had a different effect on health policy in the United States than it did in Britain. Wartime experience of military hierarchy helped create a consensus among British doctors about how medical services ought to be organized. In the United States, in contrast, similar experiences of doctors in military service further fragmented medical opinion about how to organize services. On the one hand, wartime experience stimulated the organization of group practices and the growth of medical specialties.[36] On the other, the war, in combination with the insurance crusade, persuaded many doctors that the greatest threat to their livelihoods and self-esteem would be the reorganization of medical services into efficient hierarchies.

The New Organizing Principle for Medical Services

By the end of the First World War, despite vast differences in what had been implemented, the emphasis of health policy in both nations had shifted from health to medical care. Before the second decade of the century, policy sought to promote health, a condition that could be described by laymen. After about 1920, policy was conceived mainly as providing an array of services that should be defined and evaluated by professionals who were trained in medical science.

As a result of this change in emphasis, organizing medical services became the priority of health policy in both nations. Moreover, a particular method of organizing services was, increasingly, regarded as self-evidently correct. I call this method, which I defined briefly in the Introduction, "hierarchical regionalism." The phrase is descriptive not judgmental. The word "hierarchical" describes two concepts that dominate the literature of medicine and health policy in the twentieth century. The first concept is that medical

---

[35] Richard C. Cabot, "Better Doctoring for Less Money," *American Magazine*, May 1916, 81: 43-44. *Cf.* E. A. Codman, "A Wise Preliminary to the Adoption of Any Compulsory Health Insurance Act," *Boston Medical and Surgical Journal*, March 1917, 176: 435-438, where Codman, like Cabot and Davis, took the position that no compulsory insurance was preferable to a program that did not follow the hierarchical reorganization of medical care.

[36] Stevens, *American Medicine*, 139-141.

care is work performed by people whose relative status and authority are determined by how much they know and by the complexity of the tasks they perform. The second is that these people and their workplaces should relate to each other in an orderly way that, when diagrammed, resembles a pyramid. Regionalism, as the word is used in the literature of medicine and health policy, refers to a belief that geographic areas—which may be but usually are not congruent with political jurisdictions—rather than individual practices, clinics, or hospitals, are the proper units for which to plan, administer, and evaluate medical care. Many definitions of hierarchy and regionalism have been advocated throughout the century. Each definition has embodied the views of particular individuals and groups about how medical services should be organized. Hierarchies have been proposed and created with enormous variations in formality, structure, and patterns of authority. Regions, similarly, have been proposed or created with considerable differences in size, population, and congruence with political boundaries. Thus hierarchies have been dominated by both university medical centers and free standing hospitals. Relationships within hierarchies have been described by some people as those between academics and community practitioners and by others, as those between specialists and generalists. Similarly, regions have sometimes been formally organized, by law or voluntary action, and at other times have been defined by doctors' patterns of referring patients.

This book is about what people have meant when they proposed and implemented policy to organize health services. The ponderous phrase "hierarchical regionalism" is the best one I could devise to summarize the dominant themes I found in primary sources. To put this point another way: I use the phrase because it seems to describe what most people in Britain and the United States meant when they talked about the proper way to organize health services. Moreover, the phrase summarizes what was new in twentieth-century health policy and emphasizes the events in the history of medical science and its application that were considered the justification for new policy. Hierarchical regionalism has been the framework, the preferred logic of organization, for trying to achieve important social goals. These goals include preventing and curing illness and removing financial and geographic barriers to access to services: in general, creating more rational and equitable social policies. Because the construct of hierarchical regionalism is central to my argument, I want to clarify my use of it before continuing the narrative of events in Britain and the United States.

The concept of hierarchy as I use it seems to be more readily understood than regionalism. Since the late nineteenth century, the proliferation of medical knowledge and its embodiment in technology has changed the character of institutions and the tasks of the people who worked in them. The division of labor in medical work became more complicated. Those who commanded the most sophisticated technology seemed to be almost self-evidently more important in health affairs than those whose work required less training and less investment in personnel and equipment. Unlike regionalism, hierarchy was the result of what was generally considered the progress of medicine since the nineteenth century.

Regionalism in health policy in the twentieth century, as I use the concept, differs from both earlier utopian proposals to organize the medical services in geographic areas and strategies to plan cities and stimulate regional economic growth. Regionalism has a long history as an ideal method to organize medical services. In Sir Thomas More's *Utopia*, for instance, four hospitals were located outside the walls of each city. These hospitals offered more effective medical care than the institutions of sixteenth-century England. They were "so roomy that they may pass for little towns . . . well arranged and well supplied with everything needed to cure the patients, who are nursed with tender care [and] . . . constantly attended by the most skillful physicians."[37] In the nineteenth century, Etienne Cabet in France and B. W. Richardson in Britain devised regionalized medical services for a utopian future on the basis of their faith in the progress of science. In *Icaria*, Cabet integrated hospitals, which he called the medical center of each community, with community health centers and home care.[38] In Richardson's ideal city, each district of five thousand people was served by a twenty-four bed hospital in which health services were coordinated.[39]

The concept of organizing health and social services in regions moved gradually from fantasy to policy during the nineteenth century. In both nations, sanitation and poor relief were organized on a district or metropolitan basis rather than according to existing boundaries of local government. Under the British Poor Law of 1834, aid to the deserving poor was administered in regions that were defined by socio-economic as well as political considerations. Officials of public and voluntary agencies sought to make hospital

[37] Thomas More, *Utopia* (New York: Appleton-Century-Crofts, 1949 [first published, 1516]), 39.

[38] George Rosen, "Medicine in Utopia, from the Eighteenth Century to the Present," *Ciba Symposium*, December 1945, 7: 193-195.

[39] Benjamin Ward Richardson, *Hygeia: A City of Health* (London: Macmillan, 1876), 32-36.

and outpatient services for the poor more efficient by coordinating them within geographic areas. In 1891 and 1892, for instance, a select committee of the House of Lords heard proposals to create hospital districts in London that would link general and specialized institutions and coordinate services provided under both voluntary and public auspices.[40] Similarly, in 1893, the trustees of the Boston City Hospital in Massachusetts considered and then rejected as retrogressive a proposal to build small branch hospitals. They agreed, however, to create a regional ambulance system and a network of outpatient stations.[41] A few years later, the New York State Charities Aid Association proposed to divide New York City into districts in order to facilitate the coordination of hospitals and clinics.[42]

Regionalism was also a major theme among theorists of city and economic planning in the late nineteenth and early twentieth centuries. In both countries, planners wanted the burgeoning functions of central government to be decentralized to local authorities or managers of special districts. Government and voluntary associations established regional organizations to promote economic growth in both America and Britain.[43] Many city and regional planners shared the utopian assumption that there was an ideal way to array medical services in order to restore people to health. Frederick Law Olmstead, for instance, the leading planner in the United States in the late nineteenth century, made health the criterion of urban progress since the Middle Ages.[44] Ebenezer Howard, the

[40] Select Committee of the House of Lords, *Metropolitan Hospitals*, Third Report, Session, 1892 (London: Her Majesty's Stationery Office [Hereafter HMSO], 1892), xlvi-xlvii.

[41] *Report of the Trustees of the Boston City Hospital on the Advisability of Establishing Cottage or Branch Hospitals in the Several Wards of the City* (Boston: Rockwell and Churchill, 1893), 28-31, 39-40, 42, 43; cf. Morris J. Vogel, "Machine Politics and Medical Care: The City Hospital at the Turn of the Century," in Morris J. Vogel and Charles E. Rosenberg, eds., *The Therapeutic Revolution: Essays in the Social History of American Medicine* (Philadelphia: University of Pennsylvania Press, 1979), 159-175.

[42] Phil P. Jacobs, *New Hospitals Needed in Greater New York* (New York: New York State Charities Aid Association, Publication no. 101, 1908).

[43] David Lilienthal, *TVA: Democracy on the March* (New York: Harper & Bros., 1944); Philip Selznick, *TVA and the Grass Roots* (Berkeley: University of California Press, 1949). For a survey of the literature on American social and economic regionalism see Daniel M. Fox, "Neighborhoods and Social Policy . . ." *Social Welfare Forum, 1970* (New York: Columbia University Press, 1971), 117-136; for Britain, Charles Loch Mowat, *Britain Between the Wars, 1918-1940* (Chicago: University of Chicago Press, 1955, 1969), 462-465.

[44] Jon A. Peterson, "The Impact of Sanitary Reform upon American Urban Planning, 1840-1890," *Journal of Social History*, Fall 1979, 13: 93.

British promoter of the Garden City movement, claimed that the only relevant book he remembered reading before he launched his program was Richardson's *Hygeia*.[45] Patrick Geddes, a biologist and teacher of medical students before he became a planner, believed that the proper application of science would make it possible to achieve perfect health.[46]

Regionalism in medical care had, however, only its geographic focus in common with regionalism as a method of stimulating economic growth or building more livable towns. Advocates of economic regionalism and city planning emphasized the diversity of regions and of the programs required to improve them.[47] Most proponents of regionalism in medical care, in contrast, stressed the need to maintain services of a uniform availability and quality in each region. Where economic regionalists wanted to establish unique local industries with outside capital, their counterparts in medicine emphasized distributing centralized knowledge and manpower. The goal of regionalizers of medical care was what, in the language of social policy, is called universalism; the belief that citizens should have equal access or equal entitlement to services. Economic regionalists, on the other hand, were particularists. They emphasized the differences in resources and culture that diversify production and consumption.

Nevertheless, advocates of medical and economic regionalism shared fundamental assumptions about proper social organization. For both, war was a source of example and metaphor. Both often used the lessons and language of mobilization, deployment, command, and combat to formulate and describe proposed policy. For both, moreover, the structure of industry, particularly the vertical organization of the stages of manufacturing and distributing goods, was frequently a powerful analogue. Efficiency and coordination, whether in hospitals, factories, or public works, seemed to be encouraged by large organizations whose managers exercised author-

[45] Robert Fishman, *Urban Utopias in the 20th Century: Ebenezer Howard, Frank Lloyd Wright and LeCorbusier* (New York: Basic Books, 1977), 41.

[46] Marshall Stalley, *Patrick Geddes: Spokesman for Man and the Environment* (New Brunswick: Rutgers University Press, 1972), 27, 54-55, 87-89; Anthony Sutcliffe, ed., *The Rise of Modern Urban Planning, 1800-1914* (New York: St. Martin's, 1980), 208, 210, 215; on regionalism in British government, Samuel H. Beer, *The British Political System* (New York: Random House, 1974), 62.

[47] J. D. McCallum, "The Development of British Regional Policy," in Duncan Maclennon and John B. Parr, eds., *Regional Policy: Past Experience and New Directions* (Glasgow Social and Economic Research Studies #6) (Oxford: Martin Robertson, 1979).

ity that they derived from technical knowledge. Sometimes medical science itself was used as an analogue by regional planners. Geddes, for instance, preferred medical to military or industrial metaphors. He urged planners to diagnose the problems of evolving cities and to prescribe constructive surgery for them. Most important, medical and economic regionalizers shared a belief in progress as a result of the march—in the military metaphor—of science. The purpose of regional organization had changed over a century from promoting order to facilitating change.

In the 1920s and 1930s, most of the individuals and interest groups in both countries who were concerned with health policy became committed to the method of organizing services I call hierarchical regionalism. There were, however, different emphases in each country. Most Americans accorded priority to building hospitals and arraying them in regional hierarchies. The British emphasized equity and administrative rationality when they planned hierarchies. In both countries, however, the change in the priority of health policy from replacing lost income to providing services was both a cause and a result of increased emphasis on the organization of medical care.

The new emphasis on services also changed the way individuals in both countries defined the problems of achieving greater equity in the distribution of medical care. Equity no longer meant greater access for the poor and the working class to the routine medical care provided by general practitioners. Instead the goal of greater equity was reinterpreted to reflect the logic of hierarchical regionalism. Henceforth health policy, in different ways in each country, would simultaneously address the difficult, but no longer separate, problems of organizing health services and increasing access to them.

II

Commitment to Hierarchy and Regionalism: Britain, 1918-1929

BY THE END of the First World War, social policy in Britain had become compartmentalized. Most of the people who proposed or administered social policy regarded higher wages, social and medical services, and better housing as parallel rather than competing strategies to improve the health and welfare of citizens. Advocates of new health policy gave priority to translating the results of advances in medical science into properly organized and accessible service.

People who disagreed about many details of health policy agreed about reorganizing medical services to achieve hierarchical regionalism. Leaders of each major interest group in health affairs—general practitioners, consultants, hospital trustees, medical officers of health, and civil servants—justified reorganizing medical services from their own perspective. In the years between the wars, debates about unequal access to care, about the proper roles of local authorities and voluntary associations, and about how to pay doctors increasingly took place within a context of agreement about how to organize medical services. The assumptions that governed this agreement, rather than those which caused the disagreements, gradually came to determine the allocation of resources within the health sector.

Disagreements persisted, however, within this consensus. The consensus that I emphasize would not have been evident to the many general practitioners who worried about being excluded from hospitals by consultants or losing their patients to doctors working in the clinics administered by local authorities. Medical officers of health urged that higher priority be accorded to public hospitals and home health services and to collecting and interpreting data about disease and death in the population. Hospital governors often had tense relationships with medical staffs and with officials of central and local government. Civil servants, eager to innovate or conserve, or just to rise or survive, were alternately bold and cautious amid changes in governments, ministers, and the relative power of interest groups. Nevertheless, in retrospect, the most striking characteristic of health policy in Britain after 1918 is agreement about fundamental assumptions among influential individuals and groups.

REGIONALIZATION AND THE MINISTRY OF HEALTH

The Ministry of Health, which was created in 1918, was the first result of the emerging consensus about the organization of medical care.[1] Each of the groups that shaped the mandate of the new ministry advocated regional coordination in order to promote its interests and provide the basis for coalition with competing groups. Regionalism was the political expression of a consensus that a particular form of organization would promote the progress of medicine.

The leading proponent of creating a ministry within the government was Christopher Addison, a former professor of anatomy and medical school dean who worked closely with Lloyd George in the campaign for NHI. Addison believed that the progress of medical science dictated the proper organization of medical care. Scientific research had produced new discoveries that should change what he called systems of health administration.[2] Addison looked forward to a time when "medical men [would] work in groups where for certain purposes they would combine in a common center for mutual help and have access to better means for making and confirming their diagnoses."[3]

Addison's closest ally in the Civil Service, Robert Morant, was more explicit about establishing hierarchies of medical services based on technical complexity. According to Morant, the general practitioner held the front line trenches but required support from a system of hospitals. Morant wanted this system to be public rather than voluntary. He proposed that "local health authorities have under their control a complete organization of hospitals ranging from

[1] Frank Honigsbaum, *The Struggle for the Ministry of Health*, Occasional Papers on Social Administration no. 37 (London: G. Bell, 1970).

[2] Kenneth and Jane Morgan, *The Political Career of Christopher, Viscount Addison* (Oxford: Clarendon Press, 1980).

[3] Christopher Addison, unpublished and undated memorandum in Ministry of Health Committees. Documents 1917-1918. BMA Registry, vol. 1921, London; Christopher Addison, *The Health of the People* (London: University of London Press, 1914), 8.

the cottage hospital to something approximating a full medical school . . . with motor transport as its connecting link."[4]

For his campaign to create a ministry, Addison sought allies in the insurance industry, the Conservative and Labour parties, the medical profession, and the governing boards of voluntary hospitals. He devised policies that were broad enough to offer something to each group. The basis of his coalition, however, was agreement among interest groups that the ministry would coordinate medical services in geographic areas that would not be confined by the boundaries of local governments. By the time legislation to establish a ministry was introduced late in 1918, each major party and interest group supported it.[5]

The insurance industry believed that coordination of services in regions by a ministry would protect its lucrative role in financing National Health Insurance through the voluntary associations called Approved Societies. Industry leaders feared that NHI would not be extended to cover more people and specialist hospital services if its administration were tainted with the stigma attached by public opinion to services for the poor. If all the medical services in each community were coordinated by new authorities who were supervised by the proposed ministry, a delegation of leaders told the Prime Minister and War Cabinet in 1917, the industry's fears would be allayed. These new regional authorities should be representatives of the medical profession, the public health services, and the hospitals. They should unify public hospitals and dispensaries under a single management, link public and private hospitals by voluntary agreement, and coordinate diagnostic laboratories and specialist medical services.[6] The principal author of this plan, Kingsley Wood, became Addison's parliamentary private secretary when the new ministry was formed.[7]

[4] "A Note on Sir Robert Morant's Plans for the Development of the Ministry of Health," no author, no date; but the anonymous writer claimed it was the result of discussions with Morant before his death. Public Records Office, Kew, MH 79/377. For the influence of Morant and his peers see Max Beloff, "The Whitehall Factor: The Role of the Higher Civil Service, 1919-1939" in Gillian Peele and Chris Cook, eds., *The Politics of Reappraisal, 1918-1939* (London: Macmillan, 1975).

[5] Christopher Addison, *Four and a Half Years: a Personal Diary From June, 1914 to January, 1919*, 2 vols. (London: Hutchinson and Cox., 1934), 563-564.

[6] H. Kingsley Wood, "The Ministry of Health Bill Examined and Explained," in "Scheme for a Ministry of Health and of the Functions to be Transferred to It," *National Insurance Gazette*, September 22, 1917, 6: 456-457.

[7] Frank Honigsbaum, *The Division in British Medicine* (New York: St. Martin's, 1979), 340.

A committee of Conservative-Unionist members of Parliament, led by Waldorf Astor, the publisher of the *Observer*, who would also join Addison in the new ministry, proposed that services be organized in regions that followed the boundaries of existing counties. Like the leaders of the insurance industry, Astor's committee wanted to insulate new health policy from the stigma of services for the poor. Each county medical officer should establish a hierarchy of hospitals and clinics and coordinate both public and voluntary institutions.[8]

In 1918 and 1919, the Labour party proposed a program to regionalize medical care. Addison held several confidential meetings with party officials while this program was being devised. Moreover, Morant and Addison were in frequent contact with Beatrice Webb, who served on an official committee to plan for postwar reconstruction as well as on the Labour party's Advisory Committee on Public Health.[9]

Working closely with Addison, Labour shifted its priorities from financing medical care and preventing illness to organizing services. Labour had earlier proposed nationalizing hospitals and creating a comprehensive state medical service.[10] In January 1918, a party conference resolved to nationalize the insurance industry and create what it called a unified health service for the whole community. Over the next year, however, Labour's Advisory Committee on Public Health developed a proposal to place, it said, every discovery of modern medical science within reach of all. To do this, counties should be divided into regions based on medical criteria. Services should be organized on three levels in each region. Small hospitals would be the health centers for local authorities and re-

[8] Waldorf Astor, *The Health of the People: A New National Policy* (London: Argus Printing Company, 1917), 55-62.

[9] For Addison's meetings with Labour party officials: Perry Bailie to Dr. Marian Phillipps, 25 March 1918, JSM/PH/41/123; Dr. Marian Phillipps to J. S. Middleton, 10 April 1918, JSM/PH/42; "Minutes of Deputation," 11 April 1918, File JSM/PH/44, Labour Party Archives, London. Addison joined the Labour Party in the early 1920s and served as a minister in 1929-1930 and 1945-1951.

[10] "Labour Party Conference Resolutions on Public Health," March 1929 (summarizing conferences of 1909, 1918, 1925), JSM/PH/125/1, Labour Party Archives; *cf.* Benjamin Moore, *The Dawn of the Health Age* (London: J. and A. Churchill, 1911), 180. The Labour Party, *Labour and the New Social Order: Revised in Accordance with the Resolutions of the Labour Party Conference, June 1918* (London, 1918). *Cf.* Ray Earwicker, "The Emergence of a Medical Strategy in the Labour Movement," unpublished paper read at the 1981 Conference, Society for the Social History of Medicine: *cf.* Ross McKibbon, *The Evolution of the Labour Party, 1910-1924* (London: Oxford University Press, 1974).

ceiving stations for rural areas. Two levels of more sophisticated hospitals would serve areas no larger than counties and would be linked to teaching hospitals that had national responsibilities.[11]

The coalition Addison was organizing to support a new ministry was further strengthened when the British Medical Association joined it. The BMA gave its support in exchange for assurances from Addison that, under a regional policy, general practitioners would be protected from competition with doctors who worked for local governments or who staffed the outpatient departments of teaching hospitals. In a public statement in 1918, the BMA agreed with Addison that medical science was discovering the causes of many diseases and would eventually find cures for them. The new ministry should recognize, however, that what the association called the medical forces of this country were divided into three groups—research, preventive, and clinical—each of which should be respected in a coordinated system.[12]

The BMA's definition of respect was consistent with establishing hierarchies to provide medical care. Its chief administrative officer, Dr. Alfred Cox, was an active member of the Labour Party's Advisory Committee on Public Health. The association's Hospital Committee endorsed Labour's proposal to reorganize services, asking only that the phrase "national hospitals" be changed to "teaching hospitals" and that local authorities not manage the proposed regional systems.[13] Cox told a Labour party meeting a few years later that most doctors would support a regionalized national health

[11] The Labour Party, Memorandum Prepared by the Advisory Committee on Public Health, *The Organization of the Preventive and Curative Medical Services and Hospital and Laboratory Systems Under a Ministry of Health* (London, July 1919). The committee had no difficulty, it appears, agreeing on its central recommendation on the organization of medical care: J. S. Middleton to G.D.H. Cole, May 13, 1919, JSM/PH/50, Labour Party Archives.

The significance of Labour's position should not be exaggerated. Cole, who was executive secretary of the committee, barely paid attention to health policy. See A. N. Wright, *G.D.H. Cole and Socialist Democracy* (Oxford: Clarendon Press, 1979). Moreover, a year later, in October, 1920, the Press and Publicity Sub-Committee of the party vetoed a new edition of the memorandum because of "the small sale of this pamphlet." It was, however, reprinted in 1922. Arthur Greenwood to J. S. Middleton, February 8, 1922, JSM/PH/100, Labour Party Archives. For a contrary view see Arthur Marwick, "The Labour Party and the Welfare State in Britain, 1900-1948," *American Historical Review*, December 1967, 73: 387-389.

[12] British Medical Association, *A Ministry of Health* (London: BMA, 1918), 13.

[13] British Medical Association, Hospitals Committee, Documents 1922-23. Minutes of 8 November 1922, BMA Registry, vol. 2073. The BMA Council, on February 14, 1923, asked the Hospital Committee to meet with Labour party leaders in order to bring "the hospital policy of the Association together with" the views of Labour.

service if they were convinced that it would not, in his phrase, suppress their feeling of independence.[14] Similarly, the editor of the *Lancet* was satisfied that, under a Ministry of Health, the principal hospitals would become centers of scientific medicine in their regions and would be integrated into a general medical system.[15]

Medical officers of health, doctors employed by counties and county boroughs under the Public Health Act of 1875, wanted to manage unified health services that were controlled by local authorities and coordinated by a Ministry of Health. Two former borough MOHs, Sir Arthur Newsholme and Sir George Newman, helped Addison to advocate establishing a ministry as the chief medical officers, respectively, of the Local Government Board and the Board of Education. Several MOHs proposed that curative services be organized in hierarchies. In 1916, for instance, the MOH for Gloucestershire described how he had linked general and specialist hospitals with what he called forward observation departments in order to control infectious diseases.[16]

DAWSON AND ADDISON

The most prominent doctor advocating both a new ministry and hierarchical regionalism was Bertrand [later Lord] Dawson, physician to the King since 1903 and a faculty member of the University of London. During the war, Dawson served in France as a major general. The hierarchy and teamwork of military medicine were, he discovered, a logical extension of what he had been doing for decades as an attending physician at the London Hospital. In 1918, Dawson became a public advocate of reorganizing medical services at home after the war.[17]

[14] The Labour Party, *The Hospital Problem*. The Report of a Special Conference of Labour, Hospital, Medical and Kindred Societies . . . April 28-29, 1924 (London: the Labour Party, 1924). Reprinted in *British Medical Journal Supplement*, May 3, 1924, 10. The first Labour government was in office at this time.

[15] Squire Sprigge, "Medicine and the Public," *The Cornhill Magazine*, November 1919, 47: 624-635. In *Medicine and the Public* (London: William Heineman, 1905), Sprigge did not mention coordination by levels of care. By 1919, he advocated a plan to make "the principal hospitals . . . centres of scientific medicine" linked to general practice.

[16] [J. Middleton Martin], "Extension of Institutional Medical Services," *British Medical Journal*, February 22, 1919, i: 218; J. Middleton Martin, "The Gloucestershire Scheme for the Extension of Medical Services," *The Medical Officer*, October 4, 1919: 22, 129-130.

[17] Francis Watson, *Dawson of Penn* (London: Chatto and Windus, 1950), *passim* and 142.

Reasoning from military analogies, Dawson devised a plan to link National Health Insurance and local authority health services. In two lectures on "The Future of the Medical Profession" in the summer of 1918, he proposed to reorganize medical services in new institutions. The best medicine was practiced in hospitals, where teamwork prevailed, he said. But no social class, he insisted, was adequately served by the uncoordinated hospitals of Britain. Voluntary hospitals were wholly inadequate for the masses. Middle-class people, who did not think it was right to go to a hospital, were at greater risk. Moreover, the rich, who paid famous doctors to treat them at home suffered, Dawson said, because they did not "have available to them the resources of a clinic." Hospitals should be co-ordinated with each other and with the increasingly effective preventive services, Dawson said. He urged that the best means for preserving health and curing disease be made available to every citizen. But Dawson emphasized that by "available" he did not mean free of charge. His priority was organizing, not financing, services.[18]

Dawson proposed that medical care be organized in a hierarchy that had four levels. At the highest level were teaching hospitals, which he called national institutions. The other three levels were central and local hospitals and clinics in which general practitioners would work. As in the military system he had helped to organize in France, patients should move among these levels according to explicit criteria. Dawson wanted to avoid controversy about hospitals' governance and the sources of doctors' income. He believed that voluntary hospitals and private practice should continue to exist, though managed by regional organizations coordinated in the public interest by a Ministry of Health. Doctors should, he insisted, continue to receive both fees and capitation payments, supplemented by salaries for their work in prevention.[19]

Dawson assigned prevention to the medical profession in general rather than to medical officers of health. The preventive services maintained by local authorities were becoming increasingly per-

[18] Major General Sir Bertrand Dawson, "The Future of the Medical Profession," The Cavendish Lectures, delivered July 4 and 11, 1918, *British Medical Journal*, July 13, 1918, ii: 23-26; July 20, 1918, ii: 56-60.

[19] Dawson, "The Future," *passim*. Much of the secondary literature on Dawson's influence assigns him a paramount interest in preventive medicine through the unification of curative and preventive roles. Although he began his lectures with the by then conventional reminder of the "growing appreciation" that "much disease is preventible," the burden of his argument was about personal health services.

sonal and clinical, he argued. Procedures—examination, inoculation, counseling, isolation—were replacing environmental regulation as the main tasks of public health officials. Most of these procedures ought to be performed by family doctors, who currently, he said, spent too much time diagnosing and treating illness.[20] According to Dawson, preventive procedures should logically be performed within, not apart from, regional hierarchies of practitioners and institutions.

Dawson's proposals attracted the attention of the medical and lay press at a moment when Addison's campaign for a ministry had stalled. Between April and June of 1918, the War Cabinet refused to act on a bill to create a ministry. The Local Government Board, which feared losing its authority to a Ministry of Health, wanted to substitute for it a new service, administered by local authorities, to promote maternal and child health. Lloyd George, who was preoccupied with issues of war, was opposed to launching the bill, despite Addison's advocacy.[21]

Two weeks after Dawson's lectures were published, however, Lloyd George asked Addison and Dawson to meet with him to discuss health policy.[22] The government soon introduced a bill to create a ministry. A few months later, Dawson urged Lloyd George to appoint Addison as the first minister. Early in the new year, after a general election had strengthened Lloyd George's coalition, the ministry was formally established.

Between 1919 and 1921, Addison and Dawson worked together to integrate curative and preventive services in new regional hierarchies. Addison appointed Dawson to chair a consultative council charged with recommending how medical and allied health services should be organized for the inhabitants of a particular area.[23] Addison worked cautiously to strengthen the consensus. He was eager to reorganize local health services, but he reassured the medical profession that he had no immediate plan of action and would defer consideration of policy until Dawson's council had reported.[24]

Addison faced serious political problems in Parliament, the med-

[20] Dawson, "The Future."

[21] Honigsbaum, *The Division*, 36-40.

[22] Addison, *Four and a Half Years*, 564.

[23] Ministry of Health, Consultative Council on Medical and Allied Services, *Interim Report on the Future Provision of Medical and Allied Services* (London: HMSO, 1920, Cmd. 693), 5.

[24] House of Commons, Hansard, *Parliamentary Papers*, 5th Series, vol. 116, 28 May 1919, col. 1254; cf. Christopher Addison, *Politics From Within, 1911-1918* (London: Herbert Jenkins, Ltd., 1924), for a narrative of events from Addison's point of view.

ical profession, and his own ministry, however. As minister of health, he also had responsibility for housing and thus for implementing Lloyd George's promise during the election campaign to build homes fit for heroes. But construction of new houses was delayed because of the depressed economy. Addison became a surrogate victim for right-wing adherents of the coalition government in the House of Commons who hesitated to attack Lloyd George directly.[25] Within the medical profession, both conservative general practitioners and medical officers of health worried that consultants and academic doctors would dominate the council chaired by Dawson. Moreover, Dawson antagonized the leading medical and lay civil servants in the ministry by his aggressiveness, his direct access to Addison, and his desire to relegate MOHs to subordinate status. Sir George Newman, who had outmaneuvered Newsholme to become the chief medical officer of the new ministry, challenged Dawson's assertion that Addison had authorized him to review any bill pertaining to public medical services. To Newman, Dawson and his supporters were naïve proponents of what he called the fallacy that medical policy could be made on medical criteria alone.[26]

By the time Dawson's report was published, late in 1920, Addison's political career was in decline. Within a few months, Lloyd George forced him to resign. Thus the report was published, the new minister wrote, to facilitate discussion rather than as a prospectus for immediate action.

The report recommended that medical services be reorganized according to the principles of hierarchy and regionalism. Medical knowledge, the council asserted, had far outstripped the means for its application. Medicine, it said, was not properly organized to bring advances in knowledge within reach of the people. What seemed to many people to be the most troublesome questions about health policy were, in fact, subordinate issues: how to reform the medical services for the poor, clarify the responsibilities of local governments, and expand the scope and coverage of NHI. These prob-

[25] Kenneth and Jane Morgan, *Addison; cf.* Kenneth O. Morgan, *Consensus and Disarray: The Lloyd-George Coalition Government 1918-1922* (Oxford: Clarendon Press, 1979); *cf.* Rodney Lowe, "The Erosion of State Intervention in Britain, 1917-1924," *Economic History Review*, May 1978, 31: 270-286; *cf.* Our Medical Correspondent, "Health Center," *The Times*, May 26, 1919, reporting falsely that Addison planned "to introduce a great measure dealing with medical services," which amplified medical discontent.

[26] Correspondence between Sir George Newman and Sir W. A. Robinson, June 1919, MH 73/42, PRO; *cf.* Morgan, *Addison, passim*.

lems should be solved, the council said, after the government reorganized medical services to take account of the process by which progress occurred. As a result of this increasing knowledge, the techniques for treating disease had become more complex and expensive, the report continued. Medical progress began in laboratories and teaching hospitals. This progress could be distributed properly if medical care were organized according to the levels of complexity required to prevent and treat illness, the council concluded.[27]

Addison had charged the consultative council to propose regional organizations; dominated by Dawson, it recommended organizing services in regional hierarchies, which would be managed by authorities elected by popular vote. For the first time, medical services were labeled primary and secondary. The council defined primary care as care provided in homes and doctors' offices, treatment in hospitals of twenty to forty beds, health education, and emergency, maternal and child, and environmental health services. Primary health centers, resembling in purpose and design the hospitals Richardson described in *Hygeia*, should be constructed as a focus for these services, the council said. Several primary health centers should be linked to a secondary center—a large general hospital—which should, in turn be connected with a teaching hospital and its medical school. Laboratory services, convalescent facilities—called recuperative centers by the council—and professional consultation and education should also be managed by the new regional health authorities.[28]

How services should be organized had become the starting question for health policy. Money—either to maintain the wages of members of the working class or to finance their access to services—had become a subordinate issue. As the sponsor of National Health Insurance, Lloyd George had presided over the shift in the principal purpose of health policy from maintaining income to providing medical services. Now Addison and Dawson shifted the purpose of policy once again; from providing services to the poor and the working class to specifying which services in what configuration should be available for everyone.

The council's report implied that the benefits of reorganized medical care would considerably outweigh the cost of implementing the new policy. Lord Dawson made this assumption explicit during a

[27] Ministry of Health, *Consultative Council*, 507,11.
[28] *Ibid.*, 17, 5-6, 24, 29.

meeting with private practitioners and medical officers of health in the summer of 1920. He argued that "this was not a time for criticism on the ground that the scheme would cost so many millions. What it was ultimately going to cost was of small importance."[29] Proper health policy, he said, was an open-ended commitment to provide services arrayed in the hierarchies described in the report. Medical care, as Dawson proposed to organize it, could not be measured by conventional standards of accountability. Reorganization itself had almost become a remedy for illness.

Despite their concern for autonomy, representatives of the medical profession agreed with Dawson that reorganization should be the priority of health policy. Leaders of the BMA, which spoke mainly for general practitioners, called the proposed primary centers the pivotal idea of the Dawson report.[30] Members of its Hospitals Committee, on which consultants were heavily represented, supported creating regional organizations in which patients would be referred among hospitals and suggested that doctors in central hospitals should provide advice and help at the request of doctors working in local hospitals. Moreover, the committee's statement continued, both public and voluntary hospitals should refer patients who required additional treatment and were suitable for purposes of teaching to the teaching hospitals at the apex of regional hierarchies.[31]

During the next decade, moreover, medical officers of health, became increasingly enthusiastic about the proposals of Dawson's council. Many MOHs initially resented the council's proposal to give general practitioners responsibility for preventive services in primary centers. Others criticized the council's claim that consultants should remain autonomous when they attended patients in public hospitals. But the MOHs' journal, *Public Health*, noted with approval the growing popularity of the hospital and medical services provided by the large local authorities.[32] In 1925, leaders of the

[29] "Future Provision of Medical Services: Municipal Representatives' Meeting at Bristol," *British Medical Journal*, July 17, 1920, ii: 83-86.

[30] British Medical Association, Ministry of Health Committee. Documents 1920-21. July 15, 1920. BMA Registry, vol. 2000. A contemporary historian emphasized BMA approval of the Dawson Report, quoting from the medical press: R. Westland Chalmers, *Hospitals and the State* (London: John Bale Sons and Danielson Ltd., 1928), 77.

[31] British Medical Association. Ministry of Health Committee, Documents, 1919-1920. Resolution of March 26, 1920. BMA Registry, vol. 2010, British Medical Association. Hospitals Committee, Documents, 1920-1921. Testimony to Voluntary Hospitals Commission, February 1921. BMA Registry, vol. 2005.

[32] "The Report of the Consultative Council," *Public Health*, July 1920, 33: 155, 157.

Society of MOHs told a royal commission investigating National Health Insurance that its members wanted to coordinate the restoration of health in individuals.[33] A few local authorities, Aberdeen for example, created regional hospital organizations in which patients were assigned to institutions on the basis of the complexity of their illnesses.[34] By 1929, MOHs were eager to take control of the public hospitals, built mainly in the previous century to serve the poor, because they were convinced that hospitals were the basic units of medicine, even of preventive medicine.

SIR GEORGE NEWMAN: MEDICAL CARE AS HEALTH POLICY

Sir George Newman provided a powerful rationale to MOHs throughout the 1920s and early 1930s for according priority in health policy to the organization of medical services. Newman, who had been chief medical officer of the Board of Education since 1906, was appointed CMO of the Ministry of Health in 1919, serving until 1935.[35]

Newman tried harder than anyone else in Britain or the United States during the first third of the century to develop a coherent theory of health policy. He romanticized the progress of medical science in his prolific writings and in his diaries. Moreover, like Dawson, he believed that doctors should be the primary agents in preventing the death of individuals under fifty or sixty years of age.[36] Like William Brend, moreover, he asserted that even surgery prevented disease.[37]

By 1924, Newman had rejected environmental regulation as a

---

[33] *Report of the Royal Commission on National Health Insurance* (London: HMSO, 1926, Cmd. 2596), 55-57.

[34] Political and Economic Planning, *Report on the British Health Services* (London: PEP, December 1937), 256.

[35] A first-person chronology of Newman's life is in the first volume of the six-volume *Diaries*, in the Library of the Department of Health and Social Services, London.

[36] Sir George Newman, Board of Education, *Some Notes on Medical Education in England* (London: HMSO, 1918, Cmd. 9124), 87, 117. Cf. Sir George Newman, *The Place of Public Opinion in Preventive Medicine* (London: National Health Society, 1920), 10, 21. Sir George Newman, *Health and Social Evolution* (London: George Allen and Unwin, 1931), Halley Stewart Lectures for 1930, 110, 171.

[37] Sir George Newman, Ministry of Health, *An Outline of the Practice of Preventive Medicine* (London: HMSO, 1919, Cmd. 363), 106. Despite his public enthusiasm for Dawson's proposals—an obligation thrust on him by his position as the ministry's chief medical officer—Newman disliked Dawson and his ideas. George Newman to Secretary, 14 June 1920; W. A. Robinson to Sir George Newman, 23 June 1920, Newman to Robinson, 26 June 1920; Robinson to Addison, 29 June 1920, MH 73/42, PRO.

priority in health policy in favor of hierarchical regionalism. Only medical services to individuals mattered, he insisted. This radical departure from nineteenth-century policy was, he said, a result of the discontinuity between past and present. He claimed that what he called the golden age of medicine had arrived. In the modern world, he believed, every advance in knowledge increased the potential capacity of man.[38] Like Dawson, Newman believed that advancing knowledge should be disseminated down orderly hierarchies of doctors and hospitals. But he was torn between his commitment to reorganizing medical services for individuals and his long-held belief that economic and environmental forces determined the health of populations. In 1928 he attempted a compromise. Health policy should, he concluded, place individuals in an economic position to seek more personal medical services.[39]

Throughout the 1920s and early 1930s, Newman insisted that the policies he advocated were sound because they were based on science.[40] The British people, he said, were now convinced of the success of science and clamored for its benefits.[41] Newman derived a metaphysics of health from his belief in scientific progress. Health was the solvent of social conflict: a means of proving that both class war and international war were futile and wasteful.[42] Newman continued to exude optimism about progress through medical care in the face of evidence, produced by his own staff, that high infant and maternal mortality was in large measure a result of poor nutrition linked to low wages, and that many maternal deaths in childbirth were a result of errors of medical judgment. Both infant and maternal mortality were, Newman insisted, biological problems that would be solved by medical care.[43]

Newman's career exemplified the transformation in British health policy in the early twentieth century. He had been trained in sanitation as well as in the new science of bacteriology. As a young

[38] Sir George Newman, *Public Education in Health* (London: HMSO, 1924), 4, 9, ii, 22.

[39] Sir George Newman, *Citizenship and the Survival of Civilization* (New Haven: Yale University Press, 1928), 203.

[40] Newman, *Health and Social Evolution*, 191.

[41] Sir George Newman, *The Building of a Nation's Health* (London: Macmillan and Co., 1939), 2, 165, 178.

[42] *Ibid.*, 435-436, 440.

[43] Jean Donnison, *Midwives and Medical Men* (London: Heinemann, 1977), 190-191; Jane Lewis, *The Politics of Motherhood: Child and Maternal Welfare in England, 1900-1939* (London: Croom Helm, 1980), 42-51. Charles Webster, "Healthy or Hungry Thirties," *History Workshop Journal*, Spring 1982, 5: 110-129.

official, he had shared the enthusiasm of Lloyd George for National Health Insurance to replace wages lost through illness and then worked with Robert Morant to make services rather than income the priority of the new policy.[44] He helped Addison to create a new Ministry of Health. Like Lord Dawson, he emphasized the importance of personal services, even to prevent disease, and the need to organize them in hierarchies within regions. Like most members of his generation, Newman equated scientific and social progress. He and most of his contemporaries repeatedly asserted their faith that increasing the resources allocated for medical care would reduce rates of mortality and morbidity.

THE CONSENSUS AS POLICY, 1921-1929

During the 1920s, the ideas articulated by Dawson and Newman helped to inspire policy to promote the organization of hierarchies of service in geographic regions. In 1921, just before Addison left office, he had appointed a Voluntary Hospitals Commission, chaired by Lord Cave, to propose subsidies to reduce the operating deficits that hospital leaders attributed to rising wages and inadequate government payments for the care of military casualties. In addition to proposing financial grants, the commission endorsed regionalization, though a more limited version than Dawson's council had recommended. Hospitals, the Voluntary Hospitals Commission said, should be grouped by levels as parts of a connected system. Local committees, which would be appointed by a national commission, should, it insisted, organize and grade the hospitals in each district and act as a clearinghouse for patients requiring accommodation.[45]

Officials and public commissions repeatedly endorsed reorganizing medical care by levels of technical sophistication. Throughout

[44] Newman had rejected existing British policy in private in 1911. In a "Memorandum by Sir George Newman on the National Insurance Bill," written to William Braithwaite, June 15, 1911, Newman identified personal health services and behavior, separating both of them from policy to modify the environment: "Public health is thus becoming less a matter of externals and more a question of a way of life." Braithwaite Papers, II, 78, British Library of Political and Social Science, LSE.

[45] Pertinent documents are: Ministry of Health, *Voluntary Hospitals Committee: Terms of Appointment* (London: HMSO, 1921, Cmd. 1402); Ministry of Health, *Voluntary Hospitals Committee: Final Report* (London: HMSO, 1921, Cmd. 1335); Ministry of Health, *Voluntary Hospitals Commission: Terms of Appointment* (London: HMSO, 1921, Cmd. 1402). *Cf.* Ministry of Health, Post Graduate Medical Committee, *Report of the Post Graduate Medical Committee* (London: HMSO, 1921).

the decade, governments—Coalition, Conservative, and Labour—extended the life of the Voluntary Hospitals Commission as recommended by the Cave Report. In 1925, the commission recommended that plans to group hospitals by levels of care and engage in regional planning be required before local authorities or the ministry approved new hospital construction.[46]

The Royal Commission on National Health Insurance, which reported in 1926, endorsed regional coordination leading toward a unified health service as the proper framework for the eventual extension of compulsory insurance. The majority of the commissioners, however, reasserted the purpose of health policy articulated by the Liberal government before the war. They argued that priority in spending national resources must be accorded to improving the economy. The general standard of living, they insisted, was the most important influence on the health of the country. A minority of the commissioners, however, insisted that priority in health policy be given to medical services since further improvement in the standard of health would follow the extension of medical benefits to the whole nation.[47]

The major legislation to reorganize medical care during the 1920s, the Local Government Act of 1929, demonstrated the strength of the consensus in favor of hierarchical regionalism. The act abolished the Guardians of the Poor, who were created in 1834, and permitted local authorities to convert what were called Poor Law infirmaries into public general hospitals. Officials in the Ministry of Health and the minister, Neville Chamberlain, assumed that the long-awaited repeal of the poor law would facilitate the reorganization of medical care in the best interests of the general public. Chamberlain believed that the trend of practice in modern medicine and surgery was toward establishing a hierarchy of institutions, each of which had specialized equipment and personnel. He expected the new law to encourage local officials to establish a single health authority in each area. These authorities would be responsi-

[46] Ministry of Health, *Voluntary Hospitals Commission, Interim Report* (London: HMSO, 1923); *Second Interim Report* (London: HMSO, 1924); *Final Report* (London: HMSO, 1928). The most important of this series was *Report on Voluntary Accommodation in England and Wales* (London: HMSO, 1925, Cmd. 2486) in which the commission explicitly recommended regionalization by levels of care (8).

[47] *Report* (Cmd. 2556), *passim*. The commission explicitly endorsed the recommendations of the Dawson report, citing testimony by the ministry, 55 (*cf.* vol. IV, *Minutes*, 1188-89.) A "unified health service" was endorsed on page 59, but the emphasis (62) was on services for "the poorer classes."

ble to local government but would coordinate voluntary hospitals.[48] Chamberlain reflected the considerable agreement among political and medical leaders that more medical care, provided in institutions that were arrayed according to their relative sophistication and were coordinated by regional authorities, was in the public interest.

By 1929 hierarchical regionalism had become the guiding assumption of health policy in Britain. Its validity seemed self-evident. There were, however, enormous problems of deciding how to implement it—how to organize, finance, and govern the institutions and individuals providing medical services within each region.

[48] Chamberlain declared his commitment to a "single health authority" in a memorandum of November 19, 1924 to the Cabinet; quoted in Keith Feiling, *The Life of Neville Chamberlain* (London: Macmillan, 1946, 1970), 450-460. He made his commitment explicit to Parliament in the Second Reading of the Local Government Bill of 1929: House of Commons, Hansard, *Parliamentary Debates*, 5th Series, vol. 223, 26 November 1928, col. 65ff. The ministry reasserted the commitment to hierarchical regionalism, quoting Chamberlain in Parliament, in *General Circular on the Local Government Act, 1929* (London: HMSO, 1929) 8, 13. *Cf.* David Dilks, *Neville Chamberlain*, vol. I (Cambridge: Cambridge University Press, 1984), 106-107, 328, 488-489, 568-569.

The Promise and Threat of Hierarchy: The United States, 1918-1933

IN THE UNITED STATES, as in Britain, influential individuals and groups advocated reorganizing medical services in the decade after World War I. Health politics in the two nations were, however, profoundly different. Because both general and professional politics were more centralized in Britain, interest groups worked to influence the Ministry of Health. In the United States, no single agency was an analogue of the ministry. The role of the federal government in domestic health affairs was limited to assisting the states and caring for the military, war veterans, seamen, and Indians. Although many officials of state and municipal health departments were eager to provide medical services for the poor, especially for women and children, they were easily threatened by state and county medical associations, which opposed public subsidy of diagnostic and curative services as a threat to private practice.

Such internationally respected American public health officers as Charles Chapin of Providence and Hermann N. Biggs of New York never exercised formal authority beyond state and local government, and, though they challenged doctors about the substance of practice—requiring them to report contagious diseases or criticizing improper dosage of vaccines, for example—they were usually silent about how medical care was organized. Toward the end of his career, in 1920, Biggs presumed upon his reputation as both a health officer and a private practitioner to propose that New York State establish health centers to coordinate hierarchies of medical services in rural areas where, he argued, the number of doctors was decreasing. This plan was, however, defeated as a result of lobbying by the Medical Society of New York State. A diluted version of Biggs's proposal, which was enacted in 1923, merely provided a state subsidy for public hospitals constructed by rural counties.[1]

---

[1] C.E.-A. Winslow, *The Life of Hermann M. Biggs* (Philadelphia: Lea and Febiger, 1929), 346ff., 368-369; *cf.* James H. Cassedy, *Charles V. Chapin and the Public Health Movement* (Cambridge: Harvard University Press, 1962).

FOUNDATIONS AND HEALTH POLICY

The closest analogue to the Ministry of Health in the United States was the philanthropic foundation. Just after the turn of the century, the foundations established by Andrew Carnegie and John D. Rockefeller began what became a generation of effort to reorganize American medicine by subsidizing research to speed the advance of science and of education to disseminate it. Over the next third of a century, the largest foundations allocated nearly half their gifts to medical institutions. In the decade after 1918 alone, foundations, through grants and the matching funds they attracted, added about $600 million to the budgets of American medical schools. The officers of foundations announced new policies and appropriations much as members of a British government introduced legislation. The foundations established committees made up of well-known doctors and scientists to advise them on policy much as the Ministry of Health did. Staff members of foundations, through public and private reports and their advice to trustees, wielded influence comparable to that of senior civil servants in Britain.[2]

During the first three decades of the twentieth century, the Americans who had the greatest influence on health policy never held public office. Unlike Christopher Addison or Lord Dawson, the most influential American doctor of the period, William H. Welch, served as an official only of voluntary associations: dean of the Johns Hopkins Medical School and a member of numerous boards and commissions established by the Rockefeller philanthropies. Where Robert Morant established his reputation as a senior civil servant, a similarly brilliant, imaginative, and abrasive American layman, Abraham Flexner, worked as an investigator and executive first for the Carnegie and then for the Rockefeller foundations. Other influential lay staff of foundations in the 1920s and early 1930s included Michael Davis and Edward Embree of the Rockefeller philanthropies and then the Rosenwald Fund, and John Kingsbury of the Milbank Memorial Fund. No single American can be compared with Sir George Newman. National roles similar to Sir George Newman's were played by Welch and Biggs as advisers to the Rockefeller foundations, Simon Flexner as director of the Rock-

---

[2] For sources on foundations see Daniel M. Fox, "Abraham Flexner's Unpublished Report: Foundations and Medical Education, 1909-1928," *Bulletin of the History of Medicine*, Winter 1980, 54: 475-496. *Cf.* Barry D. Karl and Stanley N. Katz, "The American Private Philanthropic Foundation and the Public Sphere, 1890-1930," *Minerva*, 1981, 19: 236-270.

efeller Institute for Medical Research, and Richard Pearce and Alan Gregg as doctor-executives who promoted foundation policies among their colleagues.

Foundations had power and influence, but they lacked authority. Their financial power was restrained by their leaders' fear that the legislatures that chartered them would restrict their powers or tax them out of existence. In the early decades of the century, for instance, John D. Rockefeller was often vilified as a cruel exploiter of labor and consumers. A bill authorizing a federal charter to establish the Rockefeller Foundation was attacked by a Republican president of the United States and was defeated in Congress. Although Andrew Carnegie's reputation was better, Henry Pritchett, the first president of the Carnegie Foundation worried that grants that imposed conditions on universities would provoke state legislatures to restrict foundations' autonomy.[3]

Foundations financed scientific research and its dissemination in medical education and practice because their trustees and staff believed that science was a cause of progress and, perhaps more important, because medicine was a relatively uncontroversial investment. When, in the second and third decades of the century, several foundations financed studies that recommended reorganizing medical care, they provoked controversy. Their response to controversy was, almost always, to change policy or to fire staff members who refused to do so.

In 1910, placing medical education on a more scientific basis seemed to be a popular object of philanthropy. For more than a decade, the American Medical Association had been trying to force inferior schools to close in order to reduce the number of institutions competing for philanthropic support. The medical staffs of many large voluntary and municipal hospitals were eager to strengthen their ties with the medical schools favored by philanthropy. When Abraham Flexner inspected American medical schools for the Carnegie Foundation in 1909 and 1910, he was accompanied by an official of the AMA, was greeted warmly by presidents and faculty members of major universities, and was applauded by many doctors and by the press when he proposed that American medical education be based on research, as it was at Johns Hopkins. The enthusiasm of organized medicine for proposals to reform education contrasted sharply with its uneasiness about the campaign during the same years for state legislation to mandate health insurance.

[3] Fox, "Flexner's Unpublished Report," 486.

The coalition supporting the reform of medical education soon disintegrated, however, when the Rockefeller philanthropies decided to make grants to schools on the condition that they establish full-time chairs in clinical departments. Welch and the Flexner brothers, Abraham and Simon, devised the full-time plan as a logical extension of the Johns Hopkins model. Full-time basic scientists were, they argued, more productive in research and teaching. Similarly, if clinicians could be relieved by full-time salaries of the distraction of having to practice in order to earn their living, they would make more rapid progress in improving diagnosis and treatment. Full-time plans, however, threatened to disrupt relationships among doctors in the communities surrounding medical schools. In many cities, these plans threatened the lucrative referral practices organized between the schools' department chairmen and their colleagues in the medical community. Some community doctors, antagonized by the endorsement of state-mandated health insurance by many medical school faculty members, interpreted the full-time plan as another strategy to force them to reorganize in hierarchies. Many well-established medical schools, moreover, could not afford to pay salaries to clinicians, even with foundation subsidies, and feared that they would be forced to close.[4]

Frustrated by this resistance to the full-time plan, the Rockefeller philanthropies temporarily adopted the more radical policy of establishing regional hierarchies based on medical schools. Their boards decided, on the recommendation of staff and consultants, to support only a small number of medical schools, each serving a particular geographic area. In an internal memorandum in 1919, Abraham Flexner recommended that funds be set aside to establish regional centers of medical education, research, and practice. John D. Rockefeller, Sr., initially allocated $50 million to this program. After an internal dispute among foundation executives about the propriety of funding a state university, the University of Iowa was awarded a grant to create a model of regional influence for other institutions to emulate.[5]

---

[4] *Ibid.*, 485. An important recent contribution to the history of medical education is Kenneth M. Ludmerer, *Learning to Heal* (New York: Basic Books, 1985).

[5] The dispute is discussed in *ibid.*, 487. In *An Autobiography* (New York: Simon and Schuster, 1960), 187, Flexner noted with pride that the Iowa regional model was quickly emulated—"within a few years"—in Missouri, Michigan, Minnesota, and Wisconsin. However, Flexner was uneasy about regionalism. In 1925, he wrote in *Medical Education: A Comparative Study* (New York: Macmillan, 1925) that "the profession rather than the university factor becomes stronger as the university becomes more distant" (p. 235).

The new Rockefeller strategy was violently attacked. Henry Pritchett, president of the Carnegie Foundation, worried in private that the use of philanthropic power to create, destroy, and transform major institutions would provoke a public backlash against the foundations. He told his own trustees that it was impossible to solve the problems of medical education in the United States by building up a small number of richly endowed and highly equipped medical schools.[6] N. P. Colwell, secretary of the AMA Council on Medical Education, who had accompanied Flexner on his site visits to medical schools a decade earlier, urged that Rockefeller funds be used to retrain doctors who had attended unreformed schools rather than to establish preeminent regional schools.[7] In addition, many doctors complained that closing more schools and raising admissions standards for those which remained would reduce opportunities for poor boys from rural areas to become doctors and eventually create shortages.[8] The foundations had overestimated the ability of a voluntary association, however well-financed, to set national policy for medical education.

The proposal to establish regional medical schools was, however, the first sign of a major shift in philanthropic strategy in health affairs. For the first twenty years of the century, the Rockefeller staff and trustees had behaved differently toward medicine in the United States from the way they behaved toward other causes in which they were interested. John D. Rockefeller and his principal philanthropic aide, Frederick W. Gates, were deeply influenced by the Protestant missionary tradition. They wanted to finance efforts to convert individuals and institutions to the new secular religion of applied science. For example, in 1906 they had founded the General Education Board to promote social change in the rural South by diffusing a new knowledge in order to reorganize education and, later, public health.[9] Similarly, the Rockefeller Foundation established the China Medical Board in 1915—the result of its continuing interest in both missions and medicine—in order, it said, to promote changes in the organization and substance of medical care in China.[10]

[6] Fox, "Flexner's Unpublished Report," 477-478, 485. Cf. William Allen Pusey, "Medical Education and Medical Service," *Journal of the American Medical Association*, January 4, 31; February 7, 14, 21, 1925, 84: 281-285, 365-369, 437-444, 513-515, 592-595.

[7] Fox, "Flexner's Unpublished Report," 489.

[8] Pusey, "Medical Education," 367.

[9] John Ettling, *The Germ of Laziness: Rockefeller Philanthropy and Public Health in the New South* (Cambridge: Harvard University Press, 1981).

[10] The Rockefeller Foundation, China Medical Board, *Second Annual Report*, January 1, 1916-December 31, 1916 (New York: The Foundation, 1917), 7.

After 1920, however, the leaders of the foundations became concerned with where doctors lived, how they practiced, how they maintained and renewed their skills, and how medical care should be organized to promote the diffusion of knowledge. In their grants for medical research and education in the United States before 1920, the leaders of the Rockefeller foundations had assumed that creating knowledge and teaching it to students would be sufficient to change medical practice. Doctors who lacked proper training would, the foundations' staff theorized, gradually be converted or replaced. Now they would, instead, be reorganized.

The foundations' new commitment to reorganizing medical services was evident in numerous projects begun in the early 1920s. The General Education Board, in a report on *The Distribution of Physicians*, argued that redistributing doctors from rural areas to cities was desirable because they should work in proximity to colleagues and hospitals.[11] The Rockefeller Foundation financed a study of dispensaries in New York and a model pay-clinic in a teaching hospital. Other foundations followed the lead of the Rockefeller philanthropies. The Milbank Memorial Fund sponsored urban and rural demonstrations of Hermann Biggs's proposal to integrate preventive and curative medicine in health centers. The Commonwealth Fund and the Duke Endowment promoted the construction of small rural hospitals. The Rosenwald Fund, led by Edward Embree, who had learned foundation work under Abraham Flexner at the General Education Board, sponsored research on the organization of services and gave special attention to medical care for blacks.[12]

Organized Medicine Responds

Many doctors resented the Rockefeller philanthropies' effort to reorganize medical practice by eliminating inferior schools and creating dominant regional institutions. The AMA led the resistance to the imposition of hierarchical standards. For the only time in the twentieth century, its House of Delegates demanded that all minimally qualified students should be permitted to study medicine. In 1922, moreover, the House resolved that more medical schools should be established and reaffirmed its opposition to the full-time

---

[11] Fox, "Flexner's Unpublished Report," 490-491.

[12] Publications and documents about foundation programs are in the medical and general periodical literature, in the Rare Book Room of the New York Academy of Medicine and in the Rockefeller Foundation Archives.

plan.[13] The association welcomed an attack on the General Education Board's report on the distribution of physicians by Raymond Pearl, Professor of Biometry at Johns Hopkins, even though he asserted that he could find no significant difference in local mortality rates between areas that had a physician and those with no physician at all.[14] In 1924, the president of the AMA, William Allen Pusey, complained about a conspiracy of universities and foundations to dominate education and practice. By increasing the length of education and thus raising its cost, the conspirators put it out of the reach of poor boys from rural backgrounds, he said, repeating the sentimental argument. As a result, an increasing number of areas were suffering a shortage of doctors.[15] Morris Fishbein, a prolific doctor-journalist on the AMA staff, reported that Pusey suddenly became a public figure as a result of enthusiasm about his views within the profession.[16]

The trustees and executives of the AMA and the members of its House of Delegates, were not, however, as thoroughly opposed to the changes the foundations promoted as their inflamed rhetoric suggested. Many of them were enthusiastic about the progress of medical science. Many of those who lamented the shortage of doctors in rural areas had, like Pusey himself, chosen to be urban specialists.[17] Their attacks on proposed reforms in medical education and care were always overstated. Perhaps, as politicians, they were eager to court support from the majority of doctors, who were general practitioners trained in unreformed schools and who feared that their patients might prefer younger doctors who were more familiar with new techniques.

Morris Fishbein presented the views of the AMA's leadership to both doctors and the general public. He was alternately expansive

[13] Morris Fishbein, *A History of the American Medical Association, 1847-1947* (Philadelphia: W. H. Saunders, 1947), 331.

[14] Raymond Pearl, "Distribution of Physicians in the United States: A Commentary on the Report of the General Education Board," *Journal of the American Medical Association*, April 4, 1925, 84: 1024-1028.

[15] Pusey, "Medical Education," 284, 595; William A. Pusey, "Medical Education and Medical Services: Some Further Facts and Considerations," *Journal of the American Medical Association*, May 15, 1926, 86: 1501-1508.

[16] On Pusey's fame see Fishbein, *History*.

[17] Joseph W. Mountin, Elliott H. Pennel, Georgie S. Brockett, "Location and Movement of Physicians, 1923 and 1938—Changes in Urban and Rural Totals for Established Physicians," *Public Health Reports*, February 16, 1945, 60: 173-185; *cf.* H. G. Weiskotten, "A Study of Present Tendencies in Medical Practice," *Bulletin of the Association of American Medical Colleges*, April 1928, 3: 130-151.

and restrained about the progress of medicine. On the one hand he believed that doctors would determine how to produce great men and great societies because medicine, he said, adapted all knowledge to human life.[18] On the other hand, he worried that, despite progress, the death rate among adults of middle and old age had not appreciably diminished in the past fifty years.[19] Similarly, although doctors must study the basic sciences, highly trained specialists lacked the concern of older physicians for a patient's family and job.[20] The ways of science were marvelous, said Fishbein, but increasing longevity would create new problems. Cancer, for instance, could become what he called the natural end of man.[21]

Fishbein's statements about health policy in the 1920s exemplified the willingness of many of the leaders of the profession to support a variety of innovations. He endorsed experimenting with prepaid group practice and compulsory insurance and agreed with proponents of social insurance that it was unconscionable for the United States to make no provision for the aged. Moreover, he suggested that illness among the poor might be mainly a result of lack of income rather than a lack of access to medical care. Medical care provided by philanthropy, he insisted, was no panacea for social unrest.[22]

Before 1932, Fishbein saw no inconsistency between speaking for organized medicine and regarding himself as a liberal intellectual. He was a friend of Clarence Darrow, the progressive lawyer, and of Eugene V. Debs, the aging Socialist hero, a member of the Chicago literary group that included the poet Carl Sandburg and the reporter-novelist Ben Hecht and a contributor of articles exposing medical fraud in the *American Mercury* when it was edited by H. L. Mencken and George Jean Nathan.[23]

Fishbein was a member of a loose coalition of doctors who were willing to contemplate changes in the organization of care, though not if they were financed by mandatory insurance. Many of these

[18] Morris Fishbein, "Medicine in Our Changing World," *Yale Review*, December 1928, 18: 344, 343.

[19] Morris Fishbein, "The Doctor and the State," *The Medical Profession and the Public: Currents and Countercurrents, Transactions of the College of Physicians of Philadelphia*, 1934, 4th series, 2: 100.

[20] Morris Fishbein, "Progress in Medical Science," *Doctors and Specialists* (Indianapolis: Bobbs-Merrill Co., 1930), 33.

[21] Fishbein, "Medicine in Our Changing World," 333, 334, 336.

[22] [Morris Fishbein], "The Cost of Medical Care," *Journal of the American Medical Association*, October 25, 1930, 95: 1266-1267.

[23] Fishbein, *Autobiography*, 12, 96, 99, 100-101, 118ff.

individuals had advocated more rigorous standards for medical education only a few years earlier, when the AMA and the foundations were more comfortable allies. Some members of the coalition were eager to restrict entry into specialty practice and eligibility for hospital privileges.

THE MAKING OF A COTERIE

Beginning in 1926, the members of this coalition, in collaboration with staff members of several foundations, began two studies that were intended to yield recommendations for change in medical education and practice. A Commission on Medical Education (CME) was financed jointly by the AMA and by the Carnegie, Macy, and Rockefeller Foundations. A Committee on the Costs of Medical Care (CCMC), was endorsed by the AMA and financed by eight foundations. The two groups had overlapping members. Each group defined its mission broadly.

The CME, whose members began to issue reports in 1927 and completed their work in 1931, achieved consensus about the purpose and content of public and philanthropic health policy. The goal of medical education and practice was success in the war on disease, its members said. Success would result, they continued, from proper education and health planning as well as from the continuous progress of science.[24]

The CME carefully endorsed the beliefs of diverse interest groups, sometimes to the point of inconsistency. Success in the war against disease would, for example, be achieved by well-trained physicians working in hierarchically organized institutions. But general practitioners were, somewhat lamely, reassured that success in this war would not depend on equipment, organization, numbers of health professionals, or even their knowledge of the problems involved. Since the beginning of the Depression in 1929, moreover, many doctors, worried about their falling income, had complained that there was an over-supply of practitioners. The CME agreed with them, pointing out that there was, therefore, no longer a need to discuss whether shortening the medical course or giving preference to students from rural districts would help to distribute physicians more equitably. Despite their concern for the sensitivities of community doctors, however, the members of the

[24] *Final Report of the Commission on Medical Education* (New York: The Commission, 1932), 1-10, 64.

CME acknowledged the higher prestige of academic medicine. The falling death rate since the 1880s, they reported, was entirely the result of the contributions of science to the safety and comfort of modern life.[25]

The members of the CME endorsed most of the proposals for reorganizing medical services that had been discussed in the previous two decades, but on the condition that they be implemented entirely by doctors. It approved of the change in the purpose of sickness insurance from providing cash to compensate for lost wages to subsidizing medical treatment. Treatment should be financed by a variety of methods, which would include mandatory sickness insurance, fees, and mutual benefit associations. The important lesson of the past was that the quality of any of these methods was a result of the extent to which the medical profession was responsible for administering it. Moreover, doctors and institutions, however they were paid, needed to be organized more rationally. There was only one desirable method of organization: creating, through regional planning, medical centers affiliated with universities.[26]

The CME's recommendations were modeled on contemporary British proposals. The commission quoted copiously from BMA publications of the late 1920s. Britain, its members said, offered a model of pluralism because it financed care through NHI and voluntary insurance as well as fees.

The authors of the CME's report may have regarded Britain as offering an example of how to achieve consensus among diverse groups. William Allan Pusey and Olin West, the general manager of the AMA, represented the interests of community doctors, much as the elected leaders of the BMA and Alfred Cox spoke for the majority of British doctors. Hugh Cabot, who had been a faculty member at Harvard, the dean at Michigan, and a staff member of the Mayo Clinic was, in his bearing and fierce defense of highly specialized practice, an American version of Bertrand Dawson. David Edsall, dean of the Harvard Medical School, and Hans Zinsser, Professor of Bacteriology at Harvard, represented academic medicine, much as the Regius Professors at Oxford and Cambridge and senior attending physicians and surgeons from London teaching hospitals spoke for British academics. Ray Lyman Wilbur was a man for all factions, a former president of the AMA, dean of the medical school, and president of Stanford University, and Secretary of the

---

[25] *Ibid.*, 400-401, 18, 121.
[26] *Ibid.*, 43, 20, 131.

Interior in the Hoover Administration, who chaired the simultaneous study of the costs of medical care. Like Christopher Addison in Lloyd George's Government, Wilbur was the rare doctor who had achieved stature in both general and medical politics.

In contrast to what occurred in Britain, however, the coalition that produced the CME report was soon destroyed when the same interest groups, joined by a few laymen, could not agree on the recommendations of the CCMC. Precisely why the consensus reached by the CME was destroyed within a year is a matter for conjecture. The worsening economic depression may have made the medical profession more cautious about reform. On the other hand, the recommendations of the CCMC majority for changes in financing care promised to provide many doctors, some of them for the first time, with a dependable source of income. The dogmatism of the CCMC's lay research staff and some of its lay members may have antagonized the doctors. But laymen were a minority of the committee.

On the basis of textual evidence, I suggest that the CCMC was polarized because a majority of its members blamed doctors for deficiencies that, they believed, could be remedied by hierarchical regionalism. The CCMC was dominated by the same coalition that had antagonized the profession in the debate about compulsory insurance a decade earlier: academic doctors, specialists in public health, and social scientists. This coalition again aroused the antagonism of large numbers of doctors by suggesting that their knowledge and judgment could not be trusted.

A sociological theory devised by a member of the CCMC, the concept of cultural lag, provided the majority with metaphors to explain the deficiencies of American medicine. According to William F. Ogburn of the University of Chicago, a great many people resisted institutional change based on scientific advance—became cultural laggards, he said—because they adhered to outmoded customs and habits. The members of a vanguard, who understood science and technology properly, must reduce lag in order to promote progress.[27]

Influential members of the CCMC and its staff considered themselves members of this vanguard. In earlier publications, some of them had used Ogburn's metaphors to attack the intelligence and competence of ordinary American doctors. Ogburn himself belit-

[27] For Ogburn see Richard H. Pells, *Radical Visions and American Dreams* (New York: Harper and Row, 1973).

tled doctors who, he said, like early handcraftsmen, clung to traditional individualistic practice. In 1927, in a book with an introduction signed by the five medical and lay intellectuals whose ideas dominated the CCMC majority, its staff director foreshadowed the polarization of 1932. The persistence of unnecessary sickness was, he wrote, simply a result of organizational maladjustment in the recent evolution of medicine.[28]

Two other laymen prominent in the work of the CCMC, Michael Davis and I. S. Falk, used the metaphors of the vanguard and the laggards to justify uncompromising antagonism toward doctors who opposed hierarchical regionalism by defending their autonomy as professionals or the sacredness of their relationship with patients. Davis and Falk were historical determinists. They believed that the progress of science made medical care the key to health, which they considered the basis of all improvements in the condition of the human race. Medical care would inevitably be reorganized to take account of science and technology, they asserted. Doctors would eventually practice in groups linked to hospitals that were arrayed in hierarchies according to their technical sophistication.[29] This system would be financed by prepayment by members of the public organized into groups of consumers. Medical practitioners, as Falk put it, could either be reactionaries or join with the forces of progress.[30]

Cultural lag was a convenient metaphor for the members of the CCMC who wanted to reorganize doctors and medical institutions into disciplined hierarchies.[31] The majority of the CCMC blamed

[28] Harry S. Moore, *American Medicine and the People's Health* (New York: D. Appleton, 1927), 61, 66.

[29] Davis made numerous statements of this point of view. Among the sharpest was his foreword to Henry A. Millis, *Sickness and Insurance* (Chicago: University of Chicago Press, 1937).

[30] A typical statement of Falk's fundamental views is, "The Present and Future Organization of Medicine," *Milbank Memorial Fund Quarterly*, 1934, 12: 117, 118, 121.

[31] See, for example Edgar E. Robinson and Paul C. Edwards, eds., *The Memoirs of Ray Lyman Wilbur, 1875-1949* (Palo Alto: Stanford University Press, 1960), 305, 312-313. *Cf.* Emmet M. Bay, *Medical Administration of Teaching Hospitals* (Chicago: University of Chicago Press, 1931). Arthur Viseltear, "C.E.-A. Winslow: His Era and His Contributions to Medical Care," in Charles E. Rosenberg, ed., *Healing and History* (New York: Science History Publications, 1979). I interpret Winslow and his colleagues in the CCMC majority as separating the organization from the financing of medical care and then placing higher priority on organization. Viseltear regards the CCMC majority as a vanguard that suffered because its proposals threatened the way medical care was financed. For a view similar to Viseltear's *cf.* Paul Starr, *The Transformation of American Medicine* (New York: Basic Books, 1982), 257-266. *Cf.* Lew-

American doctors for the problems of medical care on almost every page of their report. Although doctors should be the first contact between medical science and the people, many were not, the majority complained. Therefore patients needed guidance to select competent practitioners, they continued. Because many doctors claimed expertise they did not have, specialty practice should be restricted to those with special training and equipment, they insisted. Many doctors, the majority asserted, were not properly supervised when they treated patients in hospitals. To provide supervision, they declared, every city should emulate the few places that had placed at the disposal of their medical schools the public and voluntary, general and specialist, hospitals of their community.[32]

From this indictment of the lagging competence of many American doctors, the members of the majority derived their recommendations for change in the organization of medical services. They emphasized that what they called their most fundamental specific proposal was to create an orderly, hierarchical array of institutions and practitioners. This goal would be achieved by converting suitable hospitals into comprehensive health centers, each one serving a geographic area. These centers would be, in the words of the report, the keystone of satisfactory medical service. Each center would consist of a general hospital with inpatient, outpatient, and public health activities. Each center would, moreover, have branches and medical stations in its region. National policy for organizing medical care would be the sum of diverse regional arrangements created by properly trained doctors. Finally, the members of the majority recommended a method to finance medical services—prepayment—which would permit patients to be referred among units in a regional system without regard to their ability to pay for particular services.[33]

Eight doctors and the president of the Catholic Hospital Association dissented from the majority's proposal to reorganize medical services. They were offended, they said, by the tone of the majority report, by its assertion that doctors were to blame for problems that were not peculiar to medicine or medical care. The profession of

---

ellys F. Barker, "The Specialist and the General Practitioner in Relation to Teamwork in Medical Practice," *Journal of the American Association*, March 18, 1922, 78: 773-778; *cf.* Winford H. Smith, "Hospitals and Their Part in the Program of the Committee on the Costs of Medical Care," *Bulletin of the American Hospital Association*, January 1933, 7: 31-39.

[32] Committee on the Costs of Medical Care, *Medical Care for the American People* (Chicago: University of Chicago Press, 1932), 5, 43, 33, 40, 64, 66, 104.

[33] *Ibid.*, 109, 59-66.

medicine, the members of the minority asserted, was a personal service and could not adopt mass production methods without changing its character. They feared that the proposed medical centers would, in their words, establish a medical hierarchy in every community to dictate who might practice medicine there. Doctors would lose the autonomy that had stimulated them to make progress in the conquest of disease.[34]

The minority report, which was vigorously supported by the AMA and most state medical societies, rejected hierarchical regionalism in favor of the belief that individual doctors, rather than organizations, should be the fundamental units in the practice of medicine.[35] Group practices were, however, acceptable, even enviable, when, like the Mayo clinic, they charged fees for their services and did not compete to control medical practice locally or in a region. In editorials in *JAMA* and in the journals of many state medical societies, doctor-writers vented the resentment against academic doctors and social scientists that had smoldered in the profession for many years.[36] Many of the editorial writers pointed out that the same foundations that sponsored the CCMC had financed an earlier conspiracy to dominate medical schools and increase the authority of public health agencies. Hierarchical regionalism, which was the basis of consensus in Britain, where general practitioners and consultants did not compete with each other, had become an issue among adversaries in the United States.

The attack on the CCMC majority report, which began as an internal rebellion in the medical profession, was soon transformed by doctors into an uprising against any unwanted intervention by government in medical practice. Morris Fishbein, who from now on had no use for liberal intellectuals, made this exchange of enemies plain in his first editorial attacking the CCMC majority, when he identified its report with political revolution. Over the next two decades the phrase "socialized medicine" became a euphemism for interference with the autonomy of doctors who worked alone or in small groups by an academic elite of doctors and laymen who wanted to reorganize medical services and who seemed to have powerful allies in government agencies and the foundations.

[34] CCMC, *Medical Care*, 150, 152.

[35] *Ibid.*, 183.

[36] A photograph of the new Columbia University-Presbyterian Hospital building in New York City in a national magazine was captioned, "The latest substitute for the old family doctor: New York's 'socialized' super hospital." The article that accompanied it was titled, "Teamwork in Medicine," *Literary Digest*, May 16, 1925, 85: 22.

Government was a surrogate enemy. Had spokesmen for organized medicine directly attacked doctors who practiced in famous hospitals and held faculty positions in medical schools, they would have challenged the contemporary sources of medical prestige among the general public. An attack on a hierarchy that claimed to be based on science could be regarded by the public as an attack on science itself. The resulting devaluation of academic medicine might, therefore, devalue all medicine. Moreover, open warfare within the profession could erode patients' confidence in their doctors. It was better to attack the vehicle than the driver; better to complain about government authority and bureaucratic entanglement than to acknowledge that health policy was simply the means by which leading doctors proposed to translate into action their belief that medical progress should be disseminated through regional hierarchies.

The CCMC was a critical event in the history of health policy in the United States. The myth that its majority, innocent of any fault except idealism, were bullied by selfish leaders of organized medicine sustained a coterie that had enormous influence in debates about policy over the next twenty years. The fears generated in the medical profession by the majority report influenced doctors' political behavior for an even longer period. Arguments about proper policy were conducted as holy wars to establish opposing principles: hierarchy vs. autonomy; collectivism vs. individualism; coercion vs. freedom. Bargaining, negotiation, compromise—the fundamental characteristics of American politics—became anathema to many leaders of the interest groups concerned with health policy. General politicians, convinced that these groups would not accommodate to one another, often preferred inaction to making choices that would inevitably set some of their constituents against them. This political stalemate occurred, however, in a society in which there was growing agreement about the potential benefits of science applied to medical practice.

IV

Strengthening Consensus:
Britain, 1929-1939

BY 1929, local authorities, voluntary hospitals, and medical interest groups in Britain had begun to implement the consensus about health policy that had emerged since the First World War. Under the Local Government Act of 1929, county and borough authorities could transform hospitals built for the poor into general hospitals open to members of other classes. The governors of voluntary hospitals, especially the larger ones, had agreed to coordinate—or pretend to do so—with local authorities as the price of central government subsidy of their costs. The leaders of the major medical interest groups—general practitioners, consultants, and medical officers of health—repeatedly endorsed national and local policy to reorganize medical services in geographic areas dominated by hospitals.

Health policy was, however, a comparatively minor issue in national affairs during the 1930s. Governments and leaders of political parties were preoccupied with the economy and foreign affairs and, by the end of the decade, with defense. In the absence of strong leadership from the Cabinet, the Ministry of Health was a passive bureaucracy. Sir George Newman, the chief medical officer of health until he retired in 1935, wrote complacently about the inevitability of progress. The civil servants believed, as they advised Walter Elliott, the most ambitious health minister of the decade, that a program to diagnose and prevent cancer was more feasible than increasing the services or the population covered by national health insurance.[1]

THE MEDIA AND MEDICINE

British newspapers and magazines accorded low priority to health affairs during the 1930s. *The Daily Express*, perhaps the most repre-

---

[1] Minutes. Third Office Conference on the Development of Health Services, MH 79/409, PRO.

sentative national newspaper in the 1930s, published a "Health Page" sporadically and filled it mainly with articles about psychology and self-help. Occasional stories about new techniques to diagnose or cure diseases usually had foreign datelines.[2]

Picture Post, which became the leading magazine of the new photojournalism, emphasized medicine in its early issues. The first issue featured what the editors claimed to be the first full story of an operation. A nurse stood, the text said, like the votary of some cult, while the surgeon demonstrated mankind's achievement at its highest.[3] Four issues later, *Picture Post* described what it called the birth of a man. The prose described a doctor at work with forceps, the photographs a nurse holding a baby.[4]

Picture Post's coverage of medical care soon diminished, however. In a series of articles on diseases in 1939, drawings and photographs of clinical events occasionally interrupted dense prose. The editors were now cautious about medical progress, saying that the articles provided no romantic accounts, although they were intended to be reassuring.[5] A few months later, *Picture Post* photographed Thomas (Lord) Horder, physician to the King, and the most famous doctor in the country, in his Harley Street consulting room, which resembled a gentleman's study rather than a place where a scientific discipline was practiced. In the text, moreover, Horder made modest claims for medicine, telling the reporter that surely we live long enough.[6]

The British Broadcasting Corporation never featured health or medical issues in the 1930s. The BBC refused to air medical dramas at a time when American soap operas frequently glamorized doctors and medical settings. Its programming about health affairs consisted mainly of occasional talks by doctors. According to the BBC's historian, moreover, because of limits on political broadcasts, health policy was hardly ever discussed on the air.[7]

---

[2] The most frequent medical stories in the press were about crime or miraculous cures. Other British papers sampled included the *Daily Mirror*, the *Daily Herald*, the *News Chronicle*, and *News of the World*. The *Illustrated London News*, whether sampled in 1913 or 1938, was more interested in natural science than in medicine.

[3] Ritchie Calder, "Operation," *Picture Post*, October 1, 1938, 1: 31-38. *Picture Post* imitated *Life*—even its cover was a black and white photograph with a red and white border—but with cultural differences.

[4] Ritchie Calder, "The Birth of a Man," *Picture Post*, October 29, 1938, 1: 25-28, 62.

[5] John Langdon Davies, "Diseases Which Are Man's Worst Enemies: The Heart," *Picture Post*, July 22, 1939, 4: 58ff.

[6] "The King's Physician," *Picture Post*, December 2, 1939, 5: 26ff.

[7] Asa Briggs, *The History of Broadcasting in the United Kingdom*, vol. I: *The Birth of*

Only a few British films dramatized the achievements of medicine. Most documentaries about health issues, even those made by outstanding filmmakers, were rigorously didactic.[8] The documentary dramas about medicine produced by the March of Time in the United States distressed British critics, one of whom said that they blurred the distinction between fact and fiction. A writer in the *British Medical Journal* accused one March of Time film of endorsing the falsely exaggerated complexity of American medical technique.[9] Most of the few British feature films that had doctors as leading characters were comedies or stories of crime.[10] The apparent exception, *The Citadel*—so popular as a novel that it was serialized by the *Daily Express*—was financed by Metro-Goldwyn Mayer and had an American director, King Vidor.[11] Critics for mass-circulation papers routinely disparaged the numerous Hollywood films with medical heroes.[12]

In contrast to the reticence about medicine in news stories, radio programs, and films, advertisements for patent medicines encouraged consumers to be optimistic about new remedies allegedly based on science. Critics of unregulated advertising complained that it induced doctors to overprescribe and rely on palliatives and consumers to neglect their health.[13] The British Medical Association urged newspaper proprietors to restrain advertisers.[14]

Broadcasting (London: Oxford University Press, 1961), 256; vol. II: *The Golden Age of the Wireless* (London: Oxford University Press, 1965), 109, 113-114, 117; vol. III: *The War of Words* (London: Oxford University Press, 1970), 39-40; vol. IV: *Sound and Vision* (New York: Oxford University Press, 1979), 640.

[8] Rachel Lowe, *The History of the British Film, 1929-1939: Documentary and Educational Films of the 1930's* (London: George Allen and Unwin, 1979), 143-144, 153-154, 93, 176. For *March of Time* see Eric Barnouw, *Documentary* (New York: Oxford University Press, 1974), 121.

[9] "Medicine Marches On," *British Medical Journal*, January 28, 1939, i: 198. But: "It seems to us right and useful that the public should have authoritative information about the principal issues." "Men of Medicine," *The Lancet*, January 28, 1930, 1 : 221. Two years earlier, however, *The Lancet* had complained about the "extraordinary even alarming power" of the *March of Time*.

[10] Dennis Gifford, *The British Film Catalogue* (Newton Abbott: David and Charles, 1973).

[11] *Daily Express*, cited in "The Effect of an Elision," *The Lancet*, September 11, 1937, ii: 641; cf. Roy Armes, *A Critical History of British Cinema* (London: Secker and Warburg, 1978), 91-92.

[12] The *Daily Express* critic, for example, in a review on May 13, 1935, lamented having to see "another of those American hospital stories."

[13] Political and Economic Planning, *Report on the British Health Services* (London: PEP, 1937), 59; cf. PEP, *Report on the British Press* (London: PEP, 1938), 192.

[14] BMA, "The Association and Secret Remedies," *British Medical Journal, Supple-*

Philanthropists and health educators used the techniques of advertising, even though they condemned using them to sell proprietary drugs. A fund-raising advertisement for St. Bartholomew's Hospital in *The Daily Mail* in 1930, for example, presented a sentimental photograph of a nurse with a cluster of babies and a list of diseases whose decline, according to the text, exemplified the triumphs of preventive medicine.[15] Similarly, advertisements in women's magazines often warned of latent disorders that could be detected only as a result of medical attention.[16]

INNOVATIONS IN HEALTH POLICY

Most of the changes in the way British medical care was organized and financed in the 1930s were made, without attracting media attention, by officials of local authorities and voluntary hospital governors. Local authorities, especially in London and the larger county boroughs, provided hospital and clinic services to increasing numbers of people. By mid-decade, the authorities in the larger cities competed for paying patients with voluntary hospitals. At the same time, voluntary hospitals attracted more middle-class patients. Hospital services for these more affluent patients, both public and voluntary, were financed by private insurance and subsidies from employers, trade unions, and local government. In the decade before the Second World War, the income of the voluntary hospitals exceeded their expenditures, which stimulated their governors to undertake considerable construction and renovation.[17]

---

ment, October 3, 1936, ii: 182-183; October 10, 1936, ii: 194-195. *Cf.* Paul Vaughan, *Doctors' Commons: A Short History of the BMA* (London: Heinemann, 1959). Public regulation of drug advertising only began—and then only for cancer remedies—in 1939.

[15] *Daily Mail*, May 22, 1930, 17.

[16] For a comparison of media coverage see, Paul Adams, "Health and the State: British and American Public Health Policies in the Depression and World War II" (unpublished D.S.W. dissertation, University of California, Berkeley, 1979), 334. In 1936, Thomas Parran, surgeon general of the United States Public Health Service broke the taboo on public discussion of syphilis in the United States by publishing an article in *Reader's Digest*. Demand for the article in Britain was strong. Two magazines primarily for women circulated in both nations: Bernard MacFadden's *Women's Beauty and Health*, between 1902 and 1920, and *Good Housekeeping* from 1922. MacFadden's magazine had a "Special Edition for England," which appears to have been more restrained than the American edition in its coverage of medicine and surgery. *Good Housekeeping* in Britain was more determinedly oriented to household efficiency in the 1930s than was its American counterpart.

[17] Brian Abel-Smith, *The Hospitals, 1800-1948* (London: Heinemann, 1948); *cf.* Vi-

These innovations were the result of a consensus that hospitals should have the highest priority in medical care. Because of this consensus, British debate about health policy in the 1930s was usually a struggle for territory rather than an argument about priorities. General practitioners and managers of voluntary hospitals resented having to compete for patients with the clinics and hospitals of local authorities. Medical officers of health resisted pressure on local authorities to subsidize voluntary hospitals and were angered when many spokesmen for the voluntaries attempted to define coordination as merely full disclosure to them of plans to expand publicly owned facilities. But these conflicts were about money and control rather than about what should be done to reduce mortality and ameliorate suffering. Most doctors and hospital leaders agreed about what services should be provided and how they should be organized. Spokesmen for the British Medical Association, the Royal Colleges, the Society of Medical Officers of Health, and the Socialist Medical Association had more in common than in conflict when they talked about health policy.

The British Medical Association, which spoke mainly for general practitioners, had been committed to hierarchical regionalism as the basis for the organizing health services for a decade. In the early 1920s, the BMA's hospital policy had still accorded the highest priority to protecting voluntary hospitals and their medical staffs against intervention by officials of local or central government. The BMA had endorsed Lord Dawson's report but remained uneasy about its implications for organizing services. In 1925, however, the BMA changed its priorities. Protecting voluntarism, it declared, was now less important than creating effective hospital districts in which services should be planned and coordinated.[18] Four years later, the BMA proposed that local authorities take the initiative to coordinate the medical profession and voluntary hospitals.[19]

In the next few years, the BMA became more explicit about the goals to be achieved by reorganizing medical care. Proposing a "General Medical Service for the Nation" in 1930, the BMA advocated linking large and small hospitals in order to achieve what it called complete coordination of the whole medical service for the

vienne Walters, *Class Inequality and Health Care: The Origins and Impact of the National Health Service* (London: Croom Helm, 1980), 51-53.

[18] "Policy Affecting Hospitals," Hospital Committee Documents, 1925-26, vol. 2076; BMA Registry.

[19] "Revised Hospital Policy of the Association," Hospital Committee Documents, 1929-30, vol. 1824, BMA Registry.

community.[20] In 1937, the BMA refined its proposal for organizing hierarchies of hospitals. According to this revised plan, each region—defined vaguely but never coterminous with local government boundaries—should have a base hospital, preferably one associated with a medical school. Base hospitals would, the BMA declared, set the standard of hospital practice in their area and be centers for education and research. Smaller hospitals, staffed by general practitioners, would be grouped around a base hospital. Patients would be referred to the proper doctor or institution through a central bureau in each region.[21]

Individual spokesmen for general practitioners also promoted the organization of medical hierarchies based on hospitals. Alfred Cox, medical secretary of the BMA, argued that creating new roles for GPs in the health centers and small hospitals of an integrated system would prevent the erosion of general practice by specialism.[22] Unlike Cox, Henry Brackenbury, an influential theorist of general practice, wanted GPs to be aloof from hierarchies, relinquishing curative and even preventive medicine.[23] The generalist should be, in Brackenbury's phrase, a health custodian performing what he called a perfective or constructive role with patients. But Brackenbury had advocated regionalism based on teaching hospitals since 1920, when he proposed expanding Lord Dawson's plan by making secondary hospitals in large towns affiliates of medical schools.[24] In the 1930s, moreover, he agreed with Dawson that medical students should be trained to work in an integrated hierarchical system and supported a proposal to organize voluntary hospitals in regions according to the level of care they provided.[25]

The BMA tried to resolve the conflict between Cox and Brackenbury in 1938 by asserting that GPs could be both apart from and within hierarchies of institutions. GPs should advise, refer, and occasionally treat patients. The family doctor, the BMA decided,

[20] *The British Medical Association's Proposals for a General Medical Service for the Nation* (London: BMA, August, 1930), 34, 40.

[21] "Hospital Policy" [1938] in Medical Planning Commission, 1941-42, vol. 2075 [also vol. 1750], BMA Registry.

[22] Alfred Cox, *Among the Doctors* (London: Christopher Johnson, 1950), 117.

[23] Henry B. Brackenbury, *Patient and Doctor* (London: Hodder and Stoughton, 1935), 65-68, 75. Not surprisingly, Brackenbury frequently quoted Sir George Newman on the historical identity of preventive and curative medicine.

[24] "Ministry of Health Committee," Documents, 1919-1920, Motion by Dr. Brackenbury, vol. 2010, BMA Registry.

[25] British Medical Association, *Report of Committee on Medical Education* (London: BMA, July, 1934). Brackenbury chaired the committee.

should be primarily a health adviser, a student of applied biology who would coordinate for patients the resources of the many specialties that were the result of the advance of scientific knowledge.[26]

Like the BMA, the leaders of the British Hospitals Association were convinced that voluntary institutions could maintain their independence and authority within regional hierarchies. In 1935, the BHA established a Voluntary Hospitals Commission to promote its views. Before the commission heard any witnesses, its chairman, Viscount Sankey, told its members that problems of coordination could be solved only if voluntary and municipal hospitals cooperated in what he called a Hospitals Council. Most members of the commission agreed with him. The only dissenter was Henry Brackenbury, who doubted if voluntary and municipal hospital officials could be persuaded to achieve anything of consequence in joint regional organizations.[27]

Disagreeing with Brackenbury, spokesmen for doctors told the commission to endorse the integration of public and private institutions in sharply defined regions. Charles Hill, representing the BMA, declared that doctors were more concerned with the quality of services than with what agency provided them. Hospitals, he said, should be so thoroughly regionalized that public and voluntary institutions could have the same medical staff.[28] Representa-

---

[26] *A General Medical Service for the Nation* (London: BMA, 1938), 8, 10, 28-29. A similar conclusion was reached in the major public report on medical care of the decade, Department of Health for Scotland, Committee on Scottish Health Services, *Report* (Edinburgh: HMSO, 1936, Cmd. 5204), 221, 311. This interpretation differs from that of the most recent student of general practice in Britain, Frank Honigsbaum, *The Division of British Medicine* (London: Kegan Paul, 1979), 177-178 and elsewhere. Honigsbaum argued that the separation between GPs and consultants became more rigid in the decades between the wars as an "unintended effect" of the operation of the National Health Insurance Act. I argue that British doctors, including GPs, accepted the principle of hierarchy as a deduction from their beliefs about the progress and effectiveness of medical care.

[27] Proceedings, Voluntary Hospitals Commission, 1937, British Hospitals Contributory Schemes Association Papers. British Library of Political and Social Science, London School of Economics and Political Science, Meeting of 29 January, 1936, 2-3. The Sankey Report was published as British Hospitals Association, *Report of the Voluntary Hospitals Commission* (London: BHA, April 1937).

[28] Proceedings, Voluntary Hospitals Commission, May 13, 1936. Hill went on to laud the "extraordinary progress by the Municipal Hospitals." Hill went somewhat beyond his mandate, in "Draft Document to be Submitted to Voluntary Hospitals Commission. . . ." February 1936, Hospital Committee; Documents, 1936, Hospital Committee; Documents, 1935-36; vol. 1612, BMA Registry. Hill may have had this incident in mind when he wrote in his autobiography that, during the 1930s, "the profession itself had paved the way for much which followed and some doctors were

tives of the Royal Colleges took similar positions. Lord Dawson, speaking for the Royal College of Medicine, claimed that the municipal hospitals had financial resources while the voluntaries had medical knowledge. All the hospitals, he continued, should be governed by a Hospital Authority, a public corporation that would resemble the BBC.[29] To these leaders of the medical profession, how services were organized was more important than protecting voluntary hospitals in their territorial conflicts with local authority health services.

The doctors' advocacy of hierarchical regionalism could not, however, overcome the inertia of many of the governors of voluntary hospitals. A committee appointed by the BHA in 1938 to implement the Sankey Report decided at its first meeting that there was no need for prompt action.[30] Almost a year later, the committee decided that the BHA should consult with officials of the BMA and the Ministry of Health about jointly creating a hospital service for the nation.[31]

The medical Left continued to advocate hierarchical regionalism in the 1930s. The leaders of the Socialist Medical Association reaffirmed the principles adopted by the Labour party's Committee on Public Health in 1918 and 1919. Somerville Hastings, a founder of the SMA and a Member of both Parliament and the London County Council, told the Labour party Conference in 1933 that, because more sickness should be treated in hospitals in the future, local authorities supervised by the Ministry of Health should administer regionalized health centers and hospitals. The BMA's proposed regional hierarchies were out of date, Hastings complained, because the association did not adequately comprehend the importance of specialization in the fight against disease.[32] In 1936, Charles Brook

---

to be heartily sorry that it had done so." Lord Hill of Luton, *Both Sides of the Hill* (London: Heinemann, 1964), 84.

[29] Proceedings, Voluntary Hospitals Commission, July 1, 1936; 25 November 1936.

[30] British Hospitals Association. Provisional Central Council, 1937-1940. British Hospitals Contributory Schemes Association Papers, London School of Economics and Political Science. November, 1937, First Meeting. This restraint did not characterize all leaders of voluntary hospitals. An extraordinary—and untypical—example is Birmingham Hospitals Centre, *Laying the Foundation Stone of the Birmingham Hospitals Center*, October 23, 1934, Souvenir Program.

[31] British Hospitals Association, Provisional Central Council, 28 November 1938.

[32] Somerville Hastings, *The People's Health* (London: Labour Party, 1932). Hastings declared that the pamphlet was "not in any way a statement of official Labour Party Policy." But he introduced it as a resolution at the Party Conference of 1932, attacked the Executive for taking no action on his proposals at the conference of 1933, and had to settle for a "preliminary statement" of policy by a subcommittee of the Executive

of the SMA was enthusiastic about the new Columbia Presbyterian Hospital in New York because, he said, it was built as the result of the coordinated effort of a number of hospitals.[33] Testifying to the Sankey Commission, leaders of the SMA urged that public grants to promote regional integration be made to voluntary hospitals. Subordinating, if only temporarily, its commitment to a full-time salaried medical service to alliance with other doctors, the SMA urged the commission to recommend that an honorarium be paid to part-time consultants on hospital staffs.[34] A few years later, the New Fabian Research Bureau endorsed establishing hierarchies of health services administered by local authorities which, it said, should be reorganized to serve larger regions.[35]

Medical officers of health were prominent advocates of hierarchically arrayed services based on hospitals. In the 1920s and early 1930s, local authorities created widely admired hierarchies of health services in Aberdeen, Gloucestershire, and London. Only eight of the counties and the London County Council had chosen to manage hospitals by 1937. But thirty-seven of the eighty-three county boroughs had converted Poor Law Infirmaries into public general hospitals. Providing medical care to individuals had become the most visible activity of local government health services.[36]

Many MOHs in smaller local authorities, which could not afford

---

in 1934. During these efforts to have policy adopted, Hastings gradually retreated from his preference for a state medical service to defend what was, essentially, the BMA position. The 1934 conference was the last occasion on which the Labour party officially took up health policy before the war. When the party ignored the issue, the ideologues of the SMA dominated rhetoric on the Left. The Labour Party, *Reports of the 32nd; 33rd; 34th Annual Conference(s)* (London: Transport House, 1932, 1933, 1934). Ben Pimlott, *Labour and the Left in the 1930's* (Cambridge: Cambridge University Press, 1977) explains the low priority accorded to health and social policy within the Labour party in the 1930s. Arthur Marwick, "The Labour Party and the Welfare State in Britain, 1900-1948," *American Historical Review*, December 1967, 73: 380-403, regards party policy as more coherent and continuous between 1918 and 1946 than I do, but notes that, in the mid-1930s, even Hastings "seemed to share the general diffidence [in the party] about ambitious social planning."

[33] Charles Brook, "Hospitals in the Wrong Places," *The Star*, April 30, 1936, reprinted in his *Making Medical History* (London: Percy P. Buxton, 1946), 14.

[34] Socialist Medical Association Testimony. Proceedings, Voluntary Hospitals Commission, 29 July 1936.

[35] New Fabian Research Bureau, "Memorandum on Health Services," 1939C, Fabian Society Papers, Nuffield College, Oxford, J 41/1 Item 3. In J 41/4 there is a memorandum by Hastings complaining that the BMA scheme for a General Medical Service for the Nation, of 1938, did not sufficiently emphasize "specialization and teamwork in the fight against disease."

[36] Data from PEP, *Report on the British Health Service*, 250.

to establish public hospitals, continued to give priority to health education for mothers and children, to nutrition, and to environmental protection. Like the voluntary sector, which included both governors of fifty-bed cottage hospitals and advocates of sophisticated hospital cities, the public health sector was not monolithic.

Medical officers of health in the larger cities, however, frequently agreed about priorities and policies with leading consultants and with spokesmen for voluntary hospitals. The MOH for Glasgow endorsed the Sankey Commission's conclusion that beds were in short supply and its recommendation that consultants should be shared by voluntary and public hospitals within a region. Like the spokesmen for voluntary hospitals, moreover, he cautioned that a hospital region could not have rigid political boundaries.[37] His colleague in Birmingham was skeptical about planning formulas, asserting that the demand for hospital beds varied among regions.[38] Wilson Jameson, then a professor at the London School of Hygiene, organized an informal committee of medical officers and academic clinicians to discuss proposals for what he called a National Hospital Service.[39]

The consensus about the central role of hospitals was strongest in London. Using the Local Government Act of 1929, the London County Council acquired sixty-three general hospitals and thirteen related institutions that had been administered by the Guardians of the Poor: a total of 42,000 beds and 20,000 staff members. In 1928, under the Guardians, these hospitals had an overall patient census of eighty percent of their capacity; they were not even full on the busiest day in the winter of 1928-1929. Nevertheless, the London County Council was committed to hospital expansion. The MOH, Sir Frederick Menzies, asserted that the beds were, in fact, fully oc-

[37] A. S. MacGregor, "The Future Development of the Hospital System," *British Medical Journal, Supplement*, September 17, 1938, ii: 199-202.

[38] H. P. Newsholme, "Hospital Bed Accommodation," *Public Health*, December, 1932, 46: 73-77.

[39] H.M.C. Macaulay, "Reflections on the Origins of the National Hospital Scheme," *Public Health*, November 1974, 89: 1-3. An editorial, "The Future of Hospitals," *Public Health*, March 1940, 53: 115-117, placed priority on the principle that "the voluntary and general hospitals must become one general hospital service," rather than on a particular scheme.

Here I amend the thesis of Bentley B. Gilbert, *British Social Policy 1914-1939* (London: B. T. Batsford, 1970). Gilbert insisted (305) that "For most of the two decades between the wars, Britain had no coherent social policy." Yet he also argued (307) that by the "coming of the Second World War a consensus on social responsibility" had evolved outside Parliament, the press or the "men making the decisions." In public policy for medical care, matters were different.

cupied and that they were inadequate for the future because demand would increase as a result of advances in medical science and the desire of the middle class for hospital accommodation.[40]

The LCC soon reorganized its new hospital service. In 1930, it established laboratories at five regional centers.[41] A year later, the LCC grouped hospitals for financial analysis by the similarity of their caseload.[42] Within a few years, it established common standards, staffing patterns, forms, and records for its hospitals. By 1934, only eighteen percent of the patients admitted to the LCC's hospitals were paupers. Working- and middle-class patients were attracted to facilities that, according to Menzies, made available to them the latest advances in medical and surgical science.[43] Moreover, by 1934 each of the London teaching hospitals, although remaining under voluntary auspices, agreed to receive referrals from one or more of the general hospitals owned by the LCC.[44]

W. Allen Daley, who succeeded Menzies as MOH after serving as his deputy, was a prominent advocate of local authority dominance of health policy and a frequent spokesman for the Society of MOHs to the central government. Like his colleagues in other large county boroughs, Daley believed that local authorities should give priority to medical services for individuals. Like them, moreover, he frequently cited Sir George Newman. Sanitary work was completed, Daley declared.[45] For Daley and many other MOHs, regulating the environment was now subordinate to providing personal health services. This new priority in local government health policy was symbolized by a change in the way the annual reports of London's Medical Officer of Health were published. After 1935, the reports were issued in separate volumes, one titled *General Public Health*

[40] London County Council, *Annual Report of the Council, 1930*, vol. IV, Part I (London: LCC, 1931) 1, 35, 46.

[41] *Ibid.*, 7.

[42] LCC, *Annual Report of the Council, 1931*, vol. IV, Part II, "Public Health—Hospital Finance" (London: LCC, 1932), *passim*.

[43] LCC, *Annual Report of the Council, 1934*, vol. IV, Part I, "Public Health" (London: LCC, 1935), 5-6.

[44] In 1931, the ministry, the University of London, and the LCC created the British Post-Graduate Hospital and Medical School at the LCC's hospital at Hammersmith. (M. D. Mackenzie, "Recent Tendencies in the Development of General Hospitals in England," *Quarterly Bulletin of the Health Organization of the League of Nations*, 1934, 3: 244. This article (220-288) is a useful study of the growth in hospital accommodations and in commitment to hierarchical regionalism.

[45] W. Allen Daley, "Problems in Hospital Administration Arising Out of the Local Government Act, 1929," *Proceedings of the Royal Society of Medicine*, September 1934, 27, Part II: 1445-1456.

Administration and another, larger and more detailed, *The Hospital and General Medical Service of the Council.*[46]

THE DILEMMA OF CHOICE

The consensus about health policy among doctors, officials of central and local government, and voluntary hospital governors was challenged in the late 1930s by Britons who advocated prevention and social reform. By the mid-1930s, despite broad agreement that health policy should emphasize services to individuals, considerable data suggested that many diseases had social and economic causes. There was, however, substantial resistance to this point of view. Politicians and the press, according to one historian, were eager to "dispel widely circulated rumours concerning an increasing tide of ill-health and malnutrition among the families of the low paid workers and the unemployed." The annual reports of the Ministry of Health, for instance, written by Newman and officials he had trained, were consistently optimistic about the improving health status of the British people.[47]

Most doctors and officials avoided choosing between personal health services and measures to promote the general welfare as priorities for health policy. Proposals to reorganize curative services routinely called for both preventive measures and improvements in the standard of living. The BMA, for instance, insisted that under its proposed General Medical Service, greater attention should be paid to the economic, social, and environmental determinants of health.[48] Somerville Hastings agreed with his colleagues in the London Labour party's Health Research Group that the three major causes of ill-health, in order of importance, were poverty, a defec-

[46] The LCC's investment in hospital rehabilitation and construction between 1930 and 1938 was 5.2 million pounds: LCC, *The Hospital Service: Future Development*, Report of the Hospital and Medical Services Committee (no. 2), 11 December 1945, 3. A history appeared in LCC, *The LCC Hospitals: A Retrospect* (London: Staples Press, 1949). Perhaps in response to the success of the LCC in attracting paying patients, the committee to coordinate voluntary hospital planning and construction, which was mandated by the Local Government Act of 1929, was a failure. According to the LCC representatives, the voluntaries "made the task extremely difficult." London Voluntary Hospitals Committee, *Joint Survey of Medical and Surgical Services in the County of London* (London: P. S. King and Son, 1933).

[47] Charles Webster, "Healthy or Hungry Thirties?" *History Workshop Journal*, Spring 1982, 5: 110-129. *Cf.* Jane Lewis, *The Politics of Motherhood* (London: Croom Helm, 1980).

[48] See note 29, above.

tive environment, and inadequate medical care. Hastings assumed that prevention would be an important task for a coordinated medical service in which increasing specialization was inevitable.[49]

A handful of people in politics, business, and the professions who considered themselves political centrists challenged the consensus that personal health services were the priority of health policy. For a few years in the late 1930s, these reformers analyzed alternative policies in order to encourage national social planning. Two groups of centrists addressed policy for medical care: "The Next Five Years" and "Political and Economic Planning." The "Next Five Years," led by Harold Macmillan, then a publisher and Conservative Member of Parliament, wanted Britain to emulate what it saw as a commitment to national planning of the New Deal in the United States. Macmillan and his colleagues wanted to extend National Health Insurance to the middle class. But they accorded higher priority to improved nutrition for the working class and the poor, because, they argued, it would reduce demand for the services paid for by health insurance.[50]

"Political and Economic Planning," the more influential of the two groups, was a loose coalition of business executives and professionals who wanted to apply the social sciences to the study of public issues. PEP struggled with priorities in a massive *Report on the British Health Services*, which it published in December 1937. The report challenged, then hesitated about, and finally affirmed the consensus that health policy should be curative, hierarchical, and implemented in regions.

The authors of the PEP *Report* attempted to resolve conflicts about priorities for health policy. Because of PEP's drafting procedure, the *Report* synthesized disagreement and uncertainty. For three years, PEP circulated drafts of chapters for comment to over two hundred

[49] London Labour Party, Health Research Group, *The Public Health of London* (London: Labour Publications, Inc., 1934). The committee included Herbert Morrison, Lewis Silkin, and Alfred Salter, to name the most notable members, in addition to Hastings. Many people in the 1930s refused to consider medical care and general social policy as competing priorities in public policy. For example: Lord Horder, foreword to Richard Titmus; *Poverty and Population: A Factual Study of Contemporary Social Waste* (London: Macmillan and Co., 1938).

[50] Harold Macmillan, *The Middle Way* (London: Macmillan, 1938). *Cf.* Arthur Marwick, "Middle Opinion in the Thirties: Planning, Progress and Political 'Agreement' " *English Historical Review*, April 1964, 79: 285-298; *The Next Five Years: An Essay in Political Agreement* (London: Macmillan and Co., 1935), 184-185, 197, 200. Harold Macmillan, *Winds of Change, 1914-1939* (London: Macmillan, 1966), 634-636, lists the members of the group who drafted this manifesto.

individuals—members of every faction in medical politics except, apparently, the Socialist Medical Association. Each chapter was then revised by the PEP Health Group, a committee of doctors and laymen.[51]

Over the three years, the parts of the *Report* modified the whole. The PEP Health Group had declared its priorities unambiguously in 1934, when the project began. Better nutrition and the improvement of general practice were the principal goals of health policy, the members of the group agreed. By the time the group drafted the conclusion of the report late in 1937, however, it could no longer maintain agreement about these priorities.

The chairman of the Health Group during the first two years of its work, G. Scott Williamson, had strongly influenced the initial statement of priorities. Williamson was co-founder of the Pioneer Medical Center at Peckham, where he and his colleagues promoted health by educating families in better habits of life and especially in improved nutrition and recreation. But the staff at Peckham was also militantly conscious of potential pathology. Williamson wanted people to be examined regularly by doctors—to have what he called a health overhaul—in order to discover what he said were their cryptic diseases. He wanted general practitioners to be both health educators and specialists in diagnosis. Under his guidance, the PEP Health Group, like the staff and families at the Peckham Center, declared that prevention and health maintenance were their priorities, without fully acknowledging that they regarded diagnosis as a parallel goal.[52]

---

[51] The history of the PEP *Report*, and of the organization in the 1930s was summarized in Kenneth Lindsay, "PEP Through the 1930's: Organization, Structure, People," in John Pinder, ed., *Fifty Years of Political and Economic Planning* (London: Heinemann, 1981), 9-31. Lindsay's essay was originally written in 1961 as "Reflections on the Social and Health Services Report" in Box UP 10/5, PEP Papers, British Library of Political and Social Science, London School of Economics and Political Science. The files of the Health Group, which produced the report, begin in 1931 in PEP papers, Box WG14/2-15/3. There are allusions to early priorities scattered through the minutes for 1934; outlines of the report from the spring of 1935 accord unambiguous priority to nutrition and general practice. The absence of contact with the Socialist Medical Association, or anyone connected with the Trades Union Congress or the Labour party, is evident in the files and confirmed in Paul Addison, *The Road to 1945* (London: Jonathon Cape, 1975), 38.

[52] Williamson's strong influence is revealed in the Health Group minutes. On May 27, 1935, for example, he presented a paper on Peckham, "An Enquiry into the State of Medical Practice." For a general history of Peckham see Innes H. Pearse and G. Scott Williamson, *The Case for Action* (London: Faber and Faber, 1931) and Innes H. Pearse and L. I. Crocker, *The Peckham Experiment* (London: George Allen and Un-

Williamson was, however, outside the consensus about health policy in Britain. Most of the doctors and officials who criticized drafts of the PEP *Report* urged a significant change in its emphasis. Without denying the importance of prevention and health maintenance, they insisted that greater attention be given to the organization of services in regions based on hospitals. Because they were also uncertain about the relative importance of prevention and intervention, however, they did not directly challenge the PEP Health Group's statement of its priorities.

In response to this criticism, medical services were accorded increasing importance in successive drafts of the report. Williamson, who was distressed by the changing emphasis of the report, became estranged from the Health Group, insisting that hospital practice was the wrong focus for health policy. He had ceased to chair the group when the *Report* appeared.[53]

Nevertheless, the opening pages of the *Report* challenged the consensus among doctors, hospital leaders, and officials that providing more personal services arrayed in regional hierarchies was the priority for health policy. Instead, the *Report* demanded "first, better use and improved arrangement of existing services, second, the expansion of measures for improving nutrition . . . third, the provision of general practitioner services for dependents of insured persons . . . and fourth, increased research and information . . . on industrial and social causes of ill-health."[54] Although there was a serious shortage of hospital beds, the authors continued, hospital construction was not a priority for public policy. Regionalization should, they said, simply mean rational administration; tidying up local government boundaries and the way patients were allocated between voluntary and public systems.[55] Moreover, a policy that promoted the hierarchical organization of services would interfere with the reorientation of health services around the general practitioner in order to avoid confusion and duplication. But even in the

---

win, Ltd., 1943, 1947). *Cf.* Jane Lewis with Barbara Brooks, "The Peckham Health Centre, 'PEP,' and the Concept of General Practice During the 1930's and 1940's," *Medical History*, April 1983, 27: 151-161.

[53] Minutes of May 27, 1935, May 1, 1936, December 16, 1936. On June 4, 1937, after Williamson had left the chair, the minutes record a plunge into ambiguity from the certainties of 1935: "It was held that *probably* [my italics] a constructive nutrition policy would yield quicker returns than the extension of GP services to the dependents of insured persons." Following this vote, the group decided to send its nutrition policy for review to experts on nutrition.

[54] PEP, *Report*, 26.

[55] *Ibid.*, 18, 397.

introduction, the PEP Health Group qualified its departure from the consensus, admitting that general practitioners could not function satisfactorily unless they were supported by what it called better coordinated facilities of a more specialized nature.[56]

The authors of the *Report* were, however, uncertain about how much importance to accord to specialized medical care. "Modern developments have magnified the importance of the specialist," they asserted, "in a world in which the division of labour is one of the most potent means of advance." But specialists encroached on the work of the general practitioner and hypnotized the public. It was difficult, for example, to determine if correct diagnoses were more often the result of GPs' knowledge about their patient families and work or of the specialized scientific knowledge of consultants.[57]

Despite their uncertainty, the authors repeatedly endorsed specialization and coordination in medical care. The goal of any extension of health insurance, they insisted, was a completely planned health service, which combined general practitioners, nurses, specialists, and hospitals.[58] What GPs attempted to do must be limited because they had difficulty keeping up with the latest research. Hierarchy was an inevitable result of technical efficiency. Medical services should be regionalized and graded, the authors said, so that each patient could have access to the best practitioner.[59]

PEP's authors struggled with the contradictions between their initial statement of priorities and their endorsement of hierarchical regionalism. The absolute priority accorded to nutrition in the introduction was replaced in the conclusion by a weaker statement that it should probably have a prior claim on any funds available for extending the health services.[60] Although the nation should avoid confusing services for sickness with those required for health, general practitioners should become coordinators in a hierarchical system, just as the BMA recommended. Only the general practitioner, the authors said, could keep track of the resources of the health services on the one hand and the peculiarities and needs of individual consumers on the other.[61]

Although they were troubled by these dilemmas of choice, PEP's authors achieved insight that was unique in their generation.

[56] *Ibid.*, 25.
[57] *Ibid.*, 160-161.
[58] *Ibid.*, 222.
[59] *Ibid.*, 265-266, 312.
[60] *Ibid.*, 337.
[61] *Ibid.*, 295-397.

Health policy, current and proposed, lacked criteria for determining priorities among services. Providing more personal health services to a larger population would permit decent people to be, in their words, humane in a hard-up world. But extending services would also encourage too many resources to be allocated to patients who stirred pity and too few for prevention. The state could offset such misplaced goodwill among doctors and public officials by subsidizing individuals to bear their own curative risks—that is by providing social insurance for only a minimum set of services.[62]

The authors had moved to the edge of the consensus. They seemed about to conclude, reluctantly, that measures to promote the general welfare must take priority over policy to provide more medical services for individuals. But they retreated once again, suggesting that money could resolve ambiguity. Finance, they claimed, was the main obstacle to adopting all of their priorities.[63] Yet they knew better. If more money were available, the need to choose among priorities for policy would merely be postponed. PEP's authors realized that few people who cared about health policy in contemporary Britain wanted to confront this choice. They concluded the *Report* by eloquently but evasively asserting ambiguity about priorities. Everyone knew, they said, that such diseases as cholera, bubonic plague, malaria, and scurvy could be eliminated by improved sanitation and housing and by higher wages rather than by medical treatment. Nevertheless, everyone preferred to define the content of health policy as measures to cure and treat disease.[64]

The PEP *Report* synthesized informed opinion about health policy in the late 1930s. It affirmed the consensus that both hierarchically organized medical care and improvements in the general welfare were desirable. But it also emphasized the ambiguous relationship between these priorities. The *Report* was well received by ministers and civil servants, and it gave PEP, for the first time, national status. Eleven national and provincial newspapers explicitly supported its conclusions; forty other papers gave the *Report* prominent coverage.[65] A condensed version was published in an inexpensive paperback edition with an introduction in which Lord Horder denounced

[62] *Ibid.*, 407-409.

[63] *Ibid.*, 408.

[64] *Ibid.*, 414.

[65] Lindsay, "Reflections" and "PEP Through the 1930's"; Max Nicholson, "PEP Through the 1930's: Growth, Thinking, Performance," in Pinder, ed., *Fifty Years*, 45. Michael Young, in "The Second World War," *ibid.*, 92, said the report "foreshadowed" the National Health Service; it did, but not in the way Young implies.

as hypocrisy preaching health to the underfed. But Horder also endorsed hierarchical regionalism with the general practitioner as the coordinator—his word was "editor"—of services. It was unnecessary to choose among the goals identified in the PEP *Report*, he implied.[66] PEP had begun its analysis of health policy in order to set priorities. The result of its work was a reasoned case for tolerating ambiguity about priorities.

[66] Lord Horder, "Introduction," in S. Mervin Herbert, ed., *Britain's Health* (London: Penguin Books, 1939), xii, xvi.

V

Acrimony and Realignment:
The United States, 1932-1940

IN THE UNITED STATES in the 1930s, a consensus about the importance of medicine in the media and among people who had money to spend for health care was not translated into national health policy. The press, movies, and radio celebrated the progress of medical science and exaggerated the virtues of those who applied it. Spending for doctors and hospitals from private, philanthropic, and public sources grew. But debates about national health policy were acrimonious. Nevertheless changes in the medical profession created the basis for a new political alliance on behalf of achieving hierarchical regionalism in installments.

THE POPULARITY OF MEDICAL PROGRESS

The movies, the theater, and the press influenced perceptions of medical science and doctors. The dramatized image of medicine had changed in the 1920s. In 1913, a controversial play about venereal disease by a member of the French Academy, Eugene Brieux, had been presented in several American cities. *Damaged Goods* was about hypocrisy and personal responsibility. Brieux's doctors were powerless to treat disease; instead they made philosophical statements in order to regulate their patients' behavior.[1] By 1920, however, medical care was dramatized more optimistically. In Eugene O'Neill's play, *Anna Christie*, the heroine, unlike nineteenth-century prostitutes who wasted away from tuberculosis, instead enjoyed her stay in a hospital.[2] Similarly, Albert Cassella, whose allegorical play and movie *Death Takes A Holiday* was first produced on Broadway in 1929, invited audiences to accept the possibility that death could temporarily be postponed and suggested an analogy to hospitals.[3]

[1] Eugene Brieux, *Damaged Goods* (Philadelphia: John C. Winston Company, 1913).
[2] Eugene O'Neill, *Anna Christie* (London: Penguin Books, reprinted 1961) 28. Cf. Malcolm Goldstein, *The Political Stage: American Drama and Theater of the Great Depression* (New York: Oxford University Press, 1974), 4-5.
[3] Albert Casella, *Death Takes a Holiday* (New York: William French and Co., 1930).

The successful struggle of doctors against death was described in photographs, paintings, and films. In 1931 the photographer Edward Steichen gave the title "Death Takes a Holiday" to a photograph of surgery at the New York Postgraduate Hospital.[4] The same year, the doctor who edited the *Annals of Internal Medicine* analyzed hundreds of paintings and decided that doctors had recently become heroes in the conflict between death and medicine.[5] The most successful dramatization of enthusiasm about medicine in the 1930s was *Men in White* by Sidney Kingsley, which won the Pulitzer Prize for drama in 1933 and then became a popular movie. In staging *Men in White*, Lee Strasberg, an innovative director, sought realistic detail in operating room procedure. Like Steichen, whose photograph might have been a model for staging the play, Strasberg made surgery a ritual.[6] Similar conventions for romanticizing doctors at work were used in many films in the next few years. Films apparently influenced by *Men in White* included: *Private World, Calling Dr. Kildare, A Man to Remember, Pacific Liner, A Doctor's Story, Wife, Doctor and Nurse, The Amazing Dr. Clitterhouse*, and *The Citadel*. The standard operating room scene was satirized by the Marx brothers in *A Day at the Races*.[7] Doctors, one scholar found, were characters in over half of 800 Hollywood films in these years, but in only 25 instances were they portrayed as bad persons.[8]

In fervid prose, Paul de Kruif made doctors heroes of modern science. De Kruif published a succession of best-selling books glorifying medical science, beginning with *Microbe Hunters* in 1924.[9] He in-

---

The play was made into a movie starring Frederic March in 1934. The allegory is made explicit in Act II of the play. A character recalls seeing the face of the "Prince" (the human form assumed by Death on his holiday) in a "dream I had in a hospital . . . I was supposed to be dying." In the very next line two characters discover that roses have not withered in the three days since the "Prince" arrived.

[4] Edward Steichen, *A Life in Photography* (New York: Doubleday, 1963).

[5] Aldred Scott Warthin, *The Physician of the Dance of Death* (New York: Paul B. Hoeber, 1931), 126-127.

[6] Sidney Kingsley, *Men in White: A Play in Three Acts* (New York: Covici Friede Publishers, 1933), 85, 136. *Men in White* was the Group Theater's longest running production. *Cf.* Goldstein, *The Political Stage*, 86-87, 430-431.

[7] A list of films approved by the AMA is in "Medicine in the Movies," *Hygeia*, June 1939, 17: 486-489.

[8] John C. Burnham, "American Medicine's Golden Age: What Happened to It?" *Science*, March 19, 1982, 215: 1475, quoting a 1978 University of Minnesota dissertation, "Doctors as Hollywood Sees Them" by R. R. Malmsheimer.

[9] Notable de Kruif best sellers included *Men Against Death* (New York: Harcourt, Brace and Company, 1932) and *Health Is Wealth* (New York: Harcourt, Brace and Company, 1940). *Cf.* Charles E. Rosenberg, "Martin Arrowsmith: The Scientist as

vented or popularized phrases that were simultaneously optimistic and foreboding: for instance, "men against death," "death fighting," "the four horsemen of death," and "death's batting average." Medicine, he wrote in *The Reader's Digest* in 1941, dared to promise the transformation of human life.[10] De Kruif's journalism was the basis for such plays as Sidney Howard's *Yellowjack* and the Federal Theater Project's *Spirochete*.[11]

Many novelists were also impressed by the progress of medicine. A. J. Cronin's transatlantic best-seller, *The Citadel*, later a successful movie, described the victory of selfless doctors over their greedy colleagues.[12] In a proletarian novel, *The Hospital*, the poet Kenneth Fearing identified the success of medicine with a Marxist vision of revolution.[13] Fearing's hospital was a secular version of the institution described in Rhoda Truax's best-selling romance of 1932, in which the hero affirmed that becoming a physician was like joining a church.[14]

Photographs were a particularly compelling source of optimism about the progress of medicine. In the 1930s, new techniques of printing made it possible to reproduce photographs with unprecedented clarity on cheap paper. For the first time, books and magazines could be dominated by photographs.[15] Lawrence Stallings, in a best-selling book of 1933, *The First World War: A Photographic History*, wrote captions for photographs of doctors and patients that emphasized the horrors of war. But in most of the published photographs of the 1930s, medicine was represented as a source of optimism.[16] Such famous photographers as Margaret Bourke White, Lewis Hine, Dorothea Lange, Walker Evans, Arthur Rothstein, and

Hero," in C. E. Rosenberg, *No Other Gods* (Baltimore: Johns Hopkins University Press, 1971), 124.

[10] Paul de Kruif, "To Become a Great M.D. Begin at 14." *Reader's Digest*, June 1941, 38: 99.

[11] Goldstein, *The Political Stage*, 145, 286; Andrew Bergman, *We're in the Money: Depression America and its Films* (New York: New York University Press, 1971), 74-76; Jane de Hart Mathews, *The Federal Theater, 1935-1939: Plays, Relief, and Politics* (Princeton: Princeton University Press, 1967), 256-257.

[12] A. J. Cronin, *The Citadel* (Boston: Little, Brown and Co., 1938), 396-398.

[13] Kenneth Fearing, *The Hospital* (New York: Random House, 1939) 217, 222.

[14] Rhoda Truax, *Hospital* (New York: E. P. Dutton and Co., 1932), 299. *Cf.* Evelyn Rivers Wilbanks, "The Physician in the American Novel," *Bulletin of Bibliography*, September-December 1958, 5: 164-168.

[15] Karin Becker Ohrn, *Dorothea Lange and the Documentary Tradition* (Baton Rouge: Louisiana State University Press, 1980), 33-35; Time-Life Books, *Documentary Photography* (New York: Time Inc., 1972), 12-14, 88-89.

[16] Lawrence Stallings, *The First World War: A Photographic History* (New York: Simon & Schuster, 1933).

Paul Strand chose to perceive people, especially the poor, as grim, passive, and apprehensive, except when they smilingly received treatment from doctors or nurses.[17]

Life, the most successful magazine of photojournalism, frequently displayed and praised doctors and medical science. The first of many *Life* photoessays about medicine was impersonal; six photographs of a surgeon's gloved hands and a patient's abdomen.[18] Its first story about medical research also deemphasized individuals. "U.S. Science," the headline declared, "Wars Against an Unknown Enemy: Cancer." The most prominent photographs in this essay were of microscopic images, laboratory animals, and X-ray equipment. These photographs represented people as subordinate to technology.[19]

But *Life* soon began to publish stories of medicine emphasizing human relationships. A photo-essay on nursing mothers, in December 1936, depicted the benefits American women received from new technology.[20] Two issues later, a story celebrated Margaret Sanger and a ruling by a U.S. Court of Appeals that doctors could send contraceptives by mail.[21] Two years later, *Life* violated conventions of modesty when it published thirty-five still photographs from the March of Time film, "The Birth of a Baby."[22]

Radio conveyed optimism about the progress and promise of medical care to a larger audience than films or magazines. Patent medicine salesmen, who adapted the techniques of itinerant drug peddlers to the new medium, created mass markets for new remedies, some of them for such media-made diseases as bad breath and body odor.[23] Radio also became a source of authoritative information about medical care in the 1920s, when the American Medical Association and several philanthropic foundations began to subsi-

---

[17] The major source for the work of these photographers is the Farm Security Administration photographic collection in the Library of Congress, Washington, D.C. For a different interpretation, see John D. Stoeckle and George Abbott White, *Plain Pictures of Plain Doctoring* (Cambridge: MIT Press, 1985).

[18] "Pictures to the Editors," *Life*, January 11, 1937, 1: 62.

[19] "U.S. Science Wars Against an Unknown Enemy: Cancer," *Life*, March 1, 1937, 1: 11ff.

[20] "Mother's Milk" *Life*, December 28, 1936, 1: 22-23.

[21] "Margaret Sanger Celebrates a Birth Control Victory," *Life*, January 11, 1937, 2: 18-21.

[22] " 'The Birth of a Baby' Aims to Reduce Maternal and Infant Mortality Rates," *Life*, April 11, 1938, 4: 33-36.

[23] James G. Burrow, *AMA: Voice of American Medicine* (Baltimore: Johns Hopkins University Press, 1963), 261; Erik Barnouw, *A Tower in Babel: The History of Broadcasting to 1933* (New York: Oxford University Press, 1966), 169-171, 159; James Harvey Young, *The Medical Messiahs* (Princeton: Princeton University Press, 1967).

dize network broadcasts of medical information.[24] But radio conventions prohibited broadcasts that might stimulate listeners to imagine sex or death. In 1934, for instance, Thomas Parran, then the commissioner of health of New York State, was not permitted to use the word "syphilis" on the air.[25] Cancer was not mentioned on the radio until 1945, although a live play-by-play broadcast of surgery had been judged acceptable five years earlier.[26] Radio dramas, like movies and best-selling novels, frequently ascribed romance and glamour to medical lives. The most successful medical soap opera, "Dr. Christian," played for fifteen years to a daily audience estimated at 20 million people.[27] A committee of the AMA concluded that soap operas promoted ethical solutions to human problems.[28]

Media descriptions of doctors and medical care were cited in support of a variety of opinions about health policy. Morris Fishbein quoted *Men in White* in order to contrast selfless doctors with corrupt politicians.[29] Advocates of a comprehensive federal health program asserted in a government publication that "men in white are pushing forward the frontiers of science."[30] But the popular image of medical care was apolitical, even antipolitical: it became a factor in health policy when promoters of innovation learned to describe their proposals as above politics. Doctors fascinated the public when they appeared to be better than ordinary people.

THE GROWTH OF MEDICAL SERVICES

The health sector of the American economy grew despite the Depression. The percentage of the gross national product spent on

[24] Morris Fishbein, *An Autobiography* (New York: Doubleday, 1969) *passim*; Philip Van Ingen, *The New York Academy of Medicine: The First Hundred Years* (New York: Columbia University Press, 1949), 434-435.

[25] Bess Furman, *A Profile of the United States Public Health Service, 1789-1950* (Washington, D.C.: United States Government Printing Office, [hereafter USGPO] 1973), 398-399.

[26] *Ibid.*, 437; "The First Radio Broadcast Operation," *Life*, April 15, 1940, 8: 110.

[27] On "Dr. Christian" Philip A. Kalisch and Beatrice J. Kalisch, *The Advance of American Nursing* (Boston: Little, Brown, 1978).

[28] A survey of medical soap operas is in Raymond William Stedman, *The Serials* (Norman: University of Oklahoma Press, 1971), 340-342, 478.

[29] Morris Fishbein, "The Doctor and the State" *The Medical Profession and the Public: Currents and Cross-Currents, Transactions of the College of Physicians of Philadelphia*, 1934, 4th series, 2: 89.

[30] Interdepartmental Committee to Coordinate the Health and Welfare Activities of the Federal Government, *Toward Better National Health* (Washington, D.C.: USGPO, 1939), 4, 5.

medical care increased from 3.6 to 4.1 between 1929 and 1935.[31] Spending for doctors' services declined in the worst years of the Depression but had begun to increase again by 1934. Hospitals' income fell in 1929-1930 but soon became larger than ever before.[32] A few hospitals offered special sales on confinements and tonsillectomies.[33] Most institutions, however, regained financial stability using government and philanthropic funds and, increasingly, as a result of voluntary hospital insurance. Private gifts to hospitals in the 1930s were almost a third higher than they were in the preceding decade.[34] By 1940, fifty-six Blue Cross plans had six million subscribers.[35]

Contrary to later claims by hospital officials and a few historians, the number and distribution of American hospitals changed more sharply in the two decades after 1925 than in any comparable pe-

[31] Russell A. Nelson, "Medical Care," in John Z. Bowers and Elizabeth F. Purcell, eds., *Advances in American Medicine: Essays at the Bicentennial* (New York: Josiah Macy, Jr., Foundation, 1976), 346, arrays GNP data over time. *Cf.* U.S. Department of Commerce, *National Income and Product of the United States* (Washington, D.C.: USGPO 1951). Monroe Lerner and Odin W. Anderson, *Health Progress in the United States, 1900-1960* (Chicago: University of Chicago Press, 1963), 300, argued that ". . . consumer spending for medical care in the Depression of 1929-33 declined over 9% annually. But in each subsequent period of economic recession . . . there was actually an increase in volume and in each at a progressively higher annual rate. . . ."

[32] Lerner and Anderson, *Health Progress*, 232, argued that the depression ended for doctors by 1934. Elton Rayack, *Professional Power and American Medicine: The Economics of the AMA* (Cleveland: World Publishing Co., 1967), 73, constructed a table from data supplied in the U.S. Department of Commerce, *Survey of Current Business*, which documents that doctors' mean net income began to rise by 1934 and continued to do so thereafter.

William Weinfeld, *Income of Physicians, 1929-1949* (Washington, D.C.: United States Office of Business Economics, 1950), 10, noted that in the twenty years after 1929 the net income of doctors increased by about the same amount (approximately 109%) as the income of all wage and salary workers in the economy. But during the same years the income of doctors became substantially greater than the income of other professionals. *Cf.* Oscar W. Serbein, Jr., *Paying for Medical Care in the United States* (New York: Columbia University Press, 1953), 48. *Cf.* Malcolm T. Maceachern, "What's To Be Done About Our Empty Hospital Beds," *Hospital Management*, January 1932, 33: 192-221; Sylvia A. Law, *Blue Cross: What Went Wrong* (New Haven: Yale University Press, 1976, 2nd ed.), 6-7, on receipts and deficits.

[33] W. W. Rawson, "Hospitals in Periods of Economic Stress," *Bulletin of the American Hospital Association*, January 1932, 6: 78-83.

[34] Commission on Hospital Care, *Hospital Care in the United States* (New York: The Commonwealth Fund, 1947), 523-524.

[35] Odin W. Anderson, *Blue Cross since 1929: Accountability to the Public Trust* (Cambridge: Ballinger Publishing Co., 1975), 45; on subscribers, data compiled by C. Rufus Rorem in A. C. Bachmeyer and G. Hartman, eds., *The Hospital in Modern Society* (New York, The Commonwealth Fund, 1943), 700.

riod. General hospital beds increased by 80 percent in those years; 60 percent of this growth occurred before World War II. Moreover, 1929 was the only year in the period in which the bed-to-population ratio fell. Hospitals also became more evenly distributed during the 1930s. In 1925 only three states had four or more beds in general hospitals for each 1,000 people. By 1941, 26 more states had added enough beds to have ratios of better than 4:1000.[36]

Most hospital construction was paid for by public funds that were spent by voluntary institutions. In 1929, private investment in hospital construction slightly exceeded public; by 1939 public funds exceeded private by a ratio of four to one. The number of voluntary hospitals increased while the number under public auspice declined. Less than a quarter of the new accommodations were in federal hospitals.[37]

Americans were hospitalized in unprecedented numbers in the 1930s. In the early years of the decade, occupancy in the general hospitals owned by cities and counties increased to well over 80 percent of capacity, while rates for voluntary hospitals fell to about 60 percent and for proprietary institutions below 50 percent. By 1940, however, all types of hospitals exceeded the occupancy rates of the late 1920s. The voluntaries achieved their 1927 level in 1936 and exceeded it in each subsequent year. Proprietary hospitals attained their 1927 level by 1937.[38]

[36] This paragraph and those that follow are based on analysis of data published annually by the Council on Medical Education and Hospitals of the American Medical Association between 1906 and 1953. These data appeared in the *Journal of the American Medical Association*, titled "Hospital Service in the United States," generally in late March, but sometimes later in the spring. They revise what historians have said about medical care in the 1930s. A recent example is George Rosen, *Preventive Medicine in the United States, 1900-1975* (New York: Science History Publications, 1975), 70, who argued that in the 1930s, "few hospitals were built due to the financial difficulties of the Depression.

[37] Data for auspice is drawn from "Hospital Service in the United States," summary of chart B, 1923-1946. Data on investments in hospital construction by the private and public sectors are in the United States Department of Commerce, *Survey of Current Business* (Washington, D.C.: USGPO, 1951); Lerner and Anderson, *Health Progress*, 231, said that by the late 1930s the ratio of federal to private spending for hospital construction was 3:1. Michael Davis, "Who Finances Construction," *Modern Hospital*, November 1938, 51: 57-58, using different data sources than the Department of Commerce, concluded that there was a shift of investment from nongovernment to government sources between 1927 and 1937.

[38] "Hospital Service in the United States," summary of Chart C, 1923 [most consistent data from 1927] to 1946. The connection between investment and utilization was made explicit by research conducted in these years by staff of the United States Public Health Service: J. W. Mountin, Elliott H. Pennell, and Kay Pearson, "Factors That

Despite considerable evidence of growth, hospital leaders complained that their facilities and operating budgets did not increase quickly enough. There was widespread agreement that the men in white, in their laboratories and teaching hospitals, were solving medical problems while social arrangements for disseminating knowledge lagged behind. The superintendent of the Massachusetts General Hospital declared in 1934, for example, that the problems of American hospitals had become economic rather than medical.[39]

The most frequently cited example of the alleged lag between progress and provision was the apparent lack of beds in general hospitals. American experts adapted the nineteenth-century European standard of four beds per thousand population to contemporary conditions.[40] Between 1927 and 1935 five major studies, each using a version of this standard, concluded that the United States was under-bedded.[41] A few experts dissented from this consensus.

Influence Hospital Occupancy," *Hospitals*, March 6, 1941, 15: 18-25; "The Distribution of Hospitals and Their Financial Support in Southern States," *Southern Medical Journal*, April 1940, 33: 402-411.

[39] N. W. Faxon, "Half-Empty Hospitals," *Survey Graphic*, December 1934, 23: 604-605.

[40] The earliest published assertion of the 4:1000 ratio appears to have been by a German doctor living in London, Franz Oppert, *Hospitaler und Wohlthaetigheits-Anstalten* (Hamburg: Otto Meissner Verlag, 1859, 1872, 1879). English editions appeared with the title *Hospitals, Infirmaries and Dispensaries* (London: John Churchill and Sons, 1867, 1868, 1883). Oppert asserted that "for every thousand inhabitants the hospital ought to have four beds for the sick poor." Oppert was quoted as an authority by British authors over the next several decades. For example: J. Francis Sutherland, *Hospitals, Their History, Construction and Hygiene* (Edinburgh: E. S. Livingstone, 1882), 148-149; Frederick J. Mowat and H. Sacon Snell, *Hospital Construction and Management* (London: J. & A. Churchill, 1883), 15. The first United States mention of ratios I have found is New York Charities Aid Association, *Handbook for Hospitals*, Publication no. 32 (New York: G. P. Putnam's Sons, 1883), which urged 1:1000 in a large town. No source was given, but it was probably Henry Burdett, whose book, *Cottage Hospitals* (London: The Scientific Press, 1881, 1896) was widely read in the United States. The best source for the history of bed-planning in the United States remains Louis S. Reed and Helen Hollingsworth, *How Many General Hospital Beds Are Needed?* (United States Department of Health, Education, and Welfare, Public Health Service, Bureau of Medical Services, 1953). *Cf.* Jeanne Palmer, *Measuring Bed Needs for General Hospitals* (United States Department of Health, Education, and Welfare, Public Health Service, Division of Hospital and Medical Facilities, October, 1956, Processed). A summary table of the studies is in Paul A. Brinker and Burley Walker, "The Hill-Burton Act: 1948-1954," *Review of Economics and Statistics*, May 1962, 44: 208.

[41] Reed and Hollingsworth, *How Many*, 6-7. Trustees of the Duke Endowment, *The Small General Hospital*, Bulletin no. 3 (Charlotte: Duke Endowment, 1928, 1932). An alternative proposal for a lower rural bed ratio was presented by Alden B. Mills and Patsy Mills, "The Need for More Hospitals in Rural Areas," in *Modern Hospital*,

Two studies, for instance, concluded that increased hospital efficiency rather than more construction was the proper response to growing demand.[42] Such criticism was, however, less influential than the belief that a shortage of beds would thwart the dissemination of medical progress. By 1938 the least controversial recommendation of a Federal Interagency Committee on Health and Welfare was that the nation needed general hospital beds in the ratio of 4.6 beds per thousand persons.[43]

The immediate source of the standard of 4.6:1000 was a study prepared for the Committee on the Costs of Medical Care by Roger I. Lee, a Boston internist, and a statistician, Louis Webster Jones. Lee and Jones obtained their standard from a formula they devised on the basis of empirical evidence and judgment. Aware of the limitations of their methods, they warned readers that they used an a priori definition of adequate medical care.[44]

Lee and Jones stated a subjective standard as an equation. They estimated need by multiplying morbidity, which was recorded mainly by public hospitals and clinics, by the number of days of hospitalization that 125 prominent specialists judged to be required for each condition. Shortage or, conceivably, surplus or sufficiency,

---

March 1935, 44: 50-54. W. S. Rankin, director of the Hospital Section of the Duke Endowment, answered this argument in "How Many Surplus Beds Should the Rural Hospital Have?" *Modern Hospital*, August 1935, 45: 55-56. By 1938, Alden B. Mills had abandoned need-based ratios for a basis in demand (utilization): "How Many Beds Are Enough?" *Modern Hospital*, August 1938, 51: 55-57; Reed and Hollingsworth, *How Many*, 8, 12, 14; Michael M. Davis, "Effects of Health Insurance on Hospitals Abroad," *Bulletin of the American Hospital Association*, January 1932, 6: 47-54. Davis criticized institution-based planning in "Are There Enough Beds? Or Too Many?" *Modern Hospital*, May 1937, 48: 49-52.

[42] C. Rufus Rorem, "The Percentage of Occupancy in American Hospitals," *Journal of the American Medical Association*, June 11, 1932, 98: 2060-2062; Charles F. Neergard, "How Many Hospital Beds Are Enough?" *Journal of the American Medical Association*, March 27, 1937, 108: 1029-1033. *Cf.* Isadore Rosenfield, "Post-War Construction of Hospitals," *Hospitals*, May 1943, 17: 28-30.

[43] Technical Committee on Medical Care, Interdepartmental Committee to Coordinate Health and Welfare Activities, *The Need for a National Health Program* (Washington, D.C.: USGPO, 1938), 32.

[44] The committee described its source as simply "professional standards of adequacy." Reed and Hollingsworth (*How Many*, 14), however, asserted that "The method of arriving at this estimate was not described in the Committee's report, but it is understood that the standard used was that developed by Dr. Roger I. Lee and Lewis Webster Jones." Reed was being circumspect: he was an eyewitness to both the Lee-Jones study and the report of the Interdepartmental Committee. Roger I. Lee and Lewis Webster Jones, *The Fundamentals of Good Medical Care* (Chicago: University of Chicago Press, 1933), vii, 120, 121, 119, 14.

could be determined by subtracting either the supply of beds or the supply modified by utilization, from need.[45] If the judgments of specialists about proper length of stay for each condition reflected their behavior, the standard merely projected the demand for facilities where specialists were clustered to the rest of the nation. In fact, facilities in cities where medical schools were located met or exceeded the Lee-Jones standard in the mid-1930s: for example, in Cleveland (5.7), Cincinnati (8.4), Memphis (8.9), Los Angeles (4.9), and Syracuse (5.1).[46]

The Lee-Jones equation was a quantitative expression of shared belief. It seemed to provide an objective basis for opinions that were reinforced by the media and that were used to justify increased expenditures for hospitals during the Depression. Almost everyone—doctors, hospital managers, public officials, social scientists, and ordinary people—agreed that more medical care, using more sophisticated facilities and equipment, was urgently needed.

Toward a New Coalition

Despite this agreement, there was no New Deal for health, no innovation comparable to the policies enacted for public welfare, old-age insurance, agriculture, industry, or regional development. For the first time, however, there was extensive debate about national health policy during the 1930s. The New Deal centralized discussion of social policy, assisted by radio and national magazines. The states, which had been the focus of discussions about health policy in the past, were regarded as destined for obsolescence by many advocates of a vigorous national health policy.

Many contemporaries and most historians blamed the failure to create national health policy in the 1930s on the acrimony that had flared between 1916 and 1920 about compulsory insurance and in 1933 over the Committee on the Costs of Medical Care. Veterans of these conflicts asserted throughout the 1930s and later that national policy would be created only if an enlightened vanguard of reform defeated the entrenched power of organized medicine.

In the late 1930s a small group of doctors left the vanguard in or-

---

[45] *Ibid.*, 119 (for multiplication), 142-145, 159ff., 172ff., 300-302 (for data sources). The weakness of the morbidity data available to Lee and Jones was well known to contemporaries. Cf. Edgar Sydenstriker, "The Incidence of Various Diseases According to Age," *Public Health Reports*, May 11, 1928, 1124-1156, criticizing his own pioneering Hagerstown study.

[46] Davis, "Are There Enough Beds?" 50-51.

der to launch an alternative political strategy. The members of this emerging coalition presented themselves to the public as men in white or their emissaries who were eager to increase and disseminate scientific knowledge. They dissociated health policy from concern about poverty and social justice.

Between 1933 and 1940, however, lay men and women were the most visible advocates of new health policy. Most of them brought to their work with foundations or government agencies systematic training in research, a belief that health was the most important area of public policy, and experience in earlier conflicts with organized medicine. Many of them had advanced degrees in the social sciences: for example, Michael Davis, Walton Hamilton, C. Rufus Rorem, Bernhard J. Stern, and Louis Reed. Others were trained in the public health disciplines—bacteriology, statistics, and epidemiology; for instance, Louis Dublin, I. S. Falk, G. S. Parrott, Nathan Sinai, Edgar Sydenstriker, and C. E-A. Winslow. A few more social workers, notably John Kingsbury. The attack on the majority report of Committee on the Costs of Medical Care was a searing experience for many of these reformers. That report set their political agenda.[47]

These medical care reformers, like other New Deal intellectuals, were frequently abused in the medical and sometimes the general press and by writers of irate letters to congressmen and administration officials. But the attacks on them were more vituperative than those on intellectuals who worked in other areas of policy. Lay reformers of medical care had become surrogate targets a few years earlier. Spokesmen for organized medicine continued to be restrained by professional etiquette and respect for scientific achievement from criticizing the eminent doctors who had supported the majority of the CCMC and now looked to the New Deal to reorganize medical practice.

The lay reformers advocated ideas about health policy that had been elaborated since the first decade of the century. They assumed that health was a positive condition that could be created and en-

[47] James Rorty, *American Medicine Mobilizes* (New York: W. W. Norton and Co., 1939), 113, for Kingsbury. There is no satisfactory secondary source for the reformers. Arthur Viseltear, "C.E.-A. Winslow: His Era and His Contributions to Medical Care," in Charles E. Rosenberg, ed., *Healing and History* (New York: Science History Publications, 1979), is a useful study. Richard V. Kasius ed., *The Challenge of Facts: Selected Public Health Papers of Edgar Sydenstriker* (New York: Prodist, 1974), has a biographical introduction. Daniel M. Fox, *Economists and Health Care* (New York: Prodist, 1979), describes the economists among the reformers. Louis Dublin appears to be the only one to have published an autobiography: *After Eighty Years* (Gainesville, Fla.: University of Florida Press, 1966).

hanced primarily by medical care and only secondarily by economic growth and social justice. The attainment of health by all Americans was, however, thwarted by ignorance and greed, which they attributed, using Ogburn's metaphor, to cultural lag. In hundreds of articles and reports, the reformers insisted that the scientific knowledge and productive capacity of the United States was more advanced than its institutions.

The reformers saw themselves as members of a vanguard leading reluctant contemporaries toward proper goals. The remedies for lag seemed obvious to them, whether the laggards were the general public—the lumbering populace, in the phrase of Haven Emerson, a New York City health commissioner—or members of selfish interest groups.[48] Intellectuals who understood social trends should prescribe the future. For medical care, the remedy for lag was, as Bernhard Stern put it in a report for the Rosenwald Fund, the reorganization of both medical services and medical payment.[49]

Unlike most of the intellectuals who supported the New Deal, these reformers believed that medical care was the first priority for social reform in the United States. Michael Davis and I. S. Falk were leading advocates of this position. Davis, at this time an executive of the Rosenwald Fund, still asserted, as he had in 1920, that illness was a more important cause of poverty than either unemployment, exploitation, or lack of education. He was delighted that the goal of health insurance had changed from replacing income to providing medical services.[50] Like Davis, Falk, who worked for the Milbank Memorial Fund and then the new Social Security Administration, was convinced that the results of science, when properly disseminated, were the fundamental cause of social progress.[51]

Falk and Davis urged American politicians to emulate what Falk, misreading the evidence, described as "Lloyd-George and his small coterie [who] gave Great Britain national health insurance." Coterie

[48] Haven Emerson, "Medical Care for All of Us: The Committee on the Costs of Medical Care Reports," *Survey Graphic* (December 1932, 21: 630). Similarly, Roger Lee and Lewis Webster Jones put the onus of lag on the public rather than on physicians: "The practice of medicine cannot rise far above the cultural level of the population it serves" (*The Fundamentals*, 14).

[49] Bernhard J. Stern, *Society and Medical Progress* (Princeton: University Press, 1941), 220. *Cf.* Paul A. Dodd and E. F. Penrose, *Economic Aspects of Medical Services* (Washington, D.C.: Graphic Arts Press, 1939), 422.

[50] Michael M. Davis, "Foreword," Henry A. Millis, *Sickness and Insurance* (Chicago: University of Chicago Press, 1937).

[51] I. S. Falk, "The Present and Future Organization of Medicine," *Milbank Memorial Fund Quarterly*, 1934, 12: 117, 118, 121.

politics suited them more than Lloyd George's or Franklin D. Roosevelt's efforts to build coalitions.[52] Throughout the 1930s, Falk and Davis, in their correspondence and public activities, tried to maintain unity of purpose and program among their allies. They led numerous attacks on proposals for national health policy that did not include group practice and mandatory insurance, recruited colleagues who shared their goals for jobs in the federal government and in foundations, and used research as an instrument of reform.[53]

The vanguard led by Davis and Falk rejected invitations to join coalitions seeking incremental changes in health policy. Isaac Rubinow, for example, who now regretted his contribution to the defeat of the first campaign for health insurance, deplored younger reformers' emphasis on how medicine was organized rather than on economic security. Health policy, he now believed, should merely establish certain minimum requirements for services.[54] More important, President Franklin D. Roosevelt rejected the reformers' programs, endorsing instead social policy to provide cash benefits in simple programs. Moreover, spending public funds to build hospitals, Roosevelt told visitors who promoted the reformers' program, would be a substitute for health insurance. The federal government, he insisted, should not hinder the remarkable progress of medicine by challenging professional autonomy.[55]

The reformers tried to change the President's mind but succeeded only in isolating themselves. Davis, Falk, and Edgar Sydenstriker, another official of the Milbank Fund, advocated their program to the Committee on Economic Security, which Roosevelt appointed in 1934 to prepare his social security program. At the first meeting of the Medical Advisory Committee of the CES, Davis had an angry confrontation about health insurance with the famous neurosurgeon Harvey Cushing, who had direct access to the president. Falk and Sydenstriker wrote a staff report endorsing mandatory insurance, but then tried to prevent the advisory committee from voting on it because its defeat was assured. The staff director of the CES, Edwin Witte, an economist from the University of Wisconsin, concluded that health insurance was a subject of secondary importance

[52] Ibid., 124; cf. Fox, Economists, 21-22.

[53] I. S. Falk to Richard H. Shryock, Davis Papers, New York Academy of Medicine, M-1.

[54] I. M. Rubinow, "Do We Need Compulsory Public Health Insurance? Yes," Annals of the American Academy of Political and Social Science, November 1933, 112-113.

[55] Frances Perkins, The Roosevelt I Knew (New York: Viking Press, 1946), 282, 289, 297.

except to doctors and a few reformers. Supported by Secretary of Labor Frances Perkins, who chaired the committee and spoke for the president, Witte buried the staff report.[56]

While the vanguard advocated the CCMC majority doctrine of regional hierarchy, compulsory prepayment, and group practice to reluctant federal officials, many doctors were reconsidering their assumptions toward government funds and the organization of practice. As their receipts declined during the Depression, they became more receptive to government programs to increase the size and security of their incomes. In most states doctors accepted fees from public relief funds. The AMA Bureau of Medical Economics reported in 1934 that doctors in twenty states regarded as successful medical care programs under the Federal Emergency Relief Act.[57] Most doctors in rural areas were eager to participate in the medical care programs organized by the Resettlement (later Farm Security) Administration, which began the same year.[58] Increasing numbers of doctors received full or part-time salaries for working in hospitals, clinics, and group practices.[59] The AMA and state medical societies accepted the health provisions of the Social Security Act— grants to the states for maternal and infant care, rehabilitation of crippled children, and general public health programs.

In the early 1930s, moreover, state medical societies discussed new ways to organize and pay for care. The Medical Society of Michigan, for instance, commissioned a study of European health insurance in 1933 and a year later called for a similar program in the

[56] Edwin E. Witte, *The Development of the Social Security Act* (Madison: University of Wisconsin Press, 1962), *passim*; Edwin E. Witte, *Social Security Perspectives* (Madison: University of Wisconsin Press, 1962), 314-317. Cf. Theron F. Schlaback, *Edwin E. Witte: Cautious Reformer* (Madison: State Historical Society of Wisconsin, 1969). Cf. Daniel S. Hirshfield, *The Lost Reform: The Campaign for Compulsory Health Insurance in the United States from 1932 to 1943* (Cambridge: Harvard University Press, 1970). Cf. Paul Starr, *The Social Transformation of American Medicine* (New York: Basic Books, 1982), 266-275; cf. for a view more sympathetic to the reformers, Arthur Viseltear, "Compulsory Health Insurance and the Definition of Public Health," in Ronald L. Numbers, ed. *Compulsory Health Insurance: The Continuing American Debate* (Westport: Greenwood Press, 1982).

[57] American Medical Association, Bureau of Medical Economics, *Care of the Indigent Sick* (Chicago: AMA, 1934, 2nd ed).

[58] A contemporary source for FSA involvement was an article by Samuel Lubell and Walter Everett in the *Saturday Evening Post* that called the program "a gigantic rehearsal for health insurance." Hamilton S. Putnam, *The New Hampshire Medical Society* (Milford, N.H.: New Hampshire Medical Society, 1966), 116.

[59] The best source for public medical practice in the 1930s remains Louis Reed, *Health Insurance: The Next Step in Social Insurance* (New York: Harper and Brothers, 1937), 158-182.

United States.[60] The California Medical Association drafted a state insurance program in 1934.[61] In North Carolina, the deans of the medical schools at Duke and Chapel Hill—the latter was president of the State Medical Society—organized prepayment plans for both hospital and ambulatory care.[62] In New Hampshire, the medical society advocated group insurance against the costs of sickness.[63] Medical societies in places as different as South Carolina, Pennsylvania, Westchester County, New York, and Texas negotiated about federal and state regulations governing fees from public funds.[64]

Specialists became more assertive about how medical care should be organized and financed. The American College of Physicians, after acrimonious debate, refused either to endorse or to condemn the majority report of the Committee on the Costs of Medical Care.[65] The American College of Surgeons cautiously endorsed the principle of health insurance in 1934. Although the AMA House of Delegates condemned the surgeons for taking this position, at the same meeting it approved a ten-point health insurance platform to guide local medical societies.[66]

This growing diversity of opinion within the profession was obscured by the prominence of the American Medical Association. The AMA's authority rested on its support from state and county

[60] Burrow, *AMA*, 199.

[61] Arthur J. Viseltear, "The California Medical-Economic Survey: Paul A. Dodd vs. the California Medical Association," *Bulletin of the History of Medicine*, March-April, 1970, 44: 141-153; *cf.* Thomas N. Bonner, *Medicine in Chicago, 1850-1950* (London: Holborn Publishing Co., 1958), 215-221.

[62] Dorothy Lang, ed., *Medicine in North Carolina* (Raleigh, N.C.: The North Carolina Medical Society, 1972), 232-235.

[63] See above, note 58.

[64] *A Brief History of the South Carolina Medical Association* (Charleston, S.C.: The Association, 1948), 72-75; Howard K. Petrey, ed., *A Century of Medicine, 1848-1948: The History of the Medical Society of the State of Pennsylvania* (Harrisburg, Pa: The Society, 1952), 124; [Anonymous] *History of the Medical Society of the County of Westchester* (White Plains, N.Y.: The Society, 1947), 120; Pat Ireland Nixon, *A History of the Texas Medical Association 1853-1953* (Austin, Texas: University of Texas Press, 1953), 354-361.

[65] George M. Piersol, *Gateway of Honor: The American College of Physicians 1915-1959* (Philadelphia: The College, 1962), 93.

[66] AMA, *Digest of Official Actions* (Chicago, AMA, 1959, cited in Elton Rayack, *Professional Power*, 165-166; *cf.* Burrow, *AMA*, 235-236. On the growth of specialism during the 1930's see William D. Holden, "Graduate Medical Education" in Bowers and Purcell, *Advances in American Medicine*, 319ff. While the number of interns in hospitals almost doubled (4100 to 7219) from 1924 to 1941, the number of residents actually declined, however, (3321-3311); Chart J, "Hospital Service in the United States."

medical societies. Few doctors dared to risk losing hospital privi-leges and patients referred from colleagues by disagreeing with the views of the leaders of these societies. The AMA's House of Del-egates reinforced and led medical opinion on public issues. Its bureaucracy influenced professional opinion through journals, national meetings, and circuit-riding. AMA opinions were com-municated outside medicine by Morris Fishbein's column, which was syndicated in 250 newspapers in the mid-1930s, by pamphlets, and by educational programs in high schools. Elected officials fa-vorable to the association received political contributions. Unlike the Committee on the Costs of Medical Care, which had declined to mount a publicity campaign on the grounds that medical care should be nonpolitical, the AMA enthusiastically used the standard techniques of American politics.[67]

Political technique alone was not, however, a sufficient basis for sustaining the AMA's influence. Its leaders struggled to reflect di-verse views about proper health policy in a profession fragmented by geography and specialty. Thus, the association gradually changed its positions. In consecutive years during the 1930s the House of Delegates endorsed voluntary health insurance, increased public expenditure for medical care for the indigent and for mater-nal and child health, cash payments from public funds to citizens with disabilities, and federal subsidies for hospital construction and biomedical research.[68]

The AMA's political technique was, moreover, often inept. Con-gressmen noticed, for example, that organized medicine pressed its case despite the weak support for national health legislation from the Administration, labor unions, and farm organizations. More-over, doctor-lobbyists made such tactical errors as opposing legis-lation that had never been introduced and flooding congressional offices with identical letters poorly disguised as personal commu-nications.[69]

These errors were a consequence of deliberate oversimplification by the AMA's leaders in order to preserve the illusion of national unity in a fragmenting profession. The leaders acted as if their power would diminish if they acknowledged the diversity of opin-

[67] Edward L. Bernays, *Biography of An Idea* (New York: Simon & Schuster, 1965), 479-80.

[68] Oliver Garceau, *The Political Life of the American Medical Association* (Cambridge: Harvard University Press, 1941). *Cf.* Burrow, *AMA.*

[69] Examples of the AMA's errors of political technique are cited in Witte, *The De-velopment,* 183.

ions about health policy within the profession. They made exaggerated attacks on socialized medicine in order to rally a profession that was splitting apart. Despite its propaganda, however, the AMA accepted every proposed innovation in health policy before the end of the 1930s except mandatory insurance as consistent with its opposition to socialized medicine.

The fragmentation of medical opinion was exemplified by what presidents of state medical societies said in their annual addresses. In 1932, for example, the president of the Pennsylvania society said that he was happy to live in a golden age of medical progress. But his successor complained that the public expected too much from medicine. The next year, 1934, another Pennsylvania president attacked laymen who wanted to burden physicians with government interference, but praised the administration of medical fees by the State Emergency Relief Service.[70] A Texas president lamented overemphasis on science, stressing instead the value of doctors' human touch. Most Texas presidents, however, praised both the march of science and general practitioners who felt threatened by the academic proponents of science. Most of the presidents who praised science also feared increasing supervision of hospital practice by academic specialists.[71]

Many doctors wanted to combine the authority they derived by identifying with science and their traditional role as wise neighbors. A Kansas doctor, for example, looking backward, titled his autobiography, *Horse and Buggy Doctor*. But he had been trained in research in Berlin, was a member of the faculty of the University of Kansas Medical School, and had published more than thirty monographs and textbooks. Speaking as a scientifically trained physician, he could not recall any disease that doctors cured in nineteenth-century Kansas. But he also denounced scientific training, asserting that doctors learned medicine by experience. Dr. Hertzler's inconsistencies were, however, apparently regarded as unremarkable by a public that eagerly read his book when it was condensed in *Reader's Digest* and selected by the Book of the Month Club.[72]

Some doctors were, however, untroubled about the implications of science for practice. They saw themselves as the only members of

[70] Petry, ed., *A Century of Medicine*, 133, 153, 155-156, 158.

[71] *Nixon*, 353, 358, 363, 366, 373-374.

[72] Arthur E. Hertzler, *The Horse and Buggy Doctor* (New York: Harper and Brothers, 1938), condensed in *Reader's Digest*, September 1938, 33: 115-130. *Cf.* Arthur E. Hertzler, M.D., *Surgical Pathology of the Diseases of the Bone* (Philadelphia: 1930).

the profession who were entitled to be revered as men in white. This group consisted mainly of the academic doctors who had been the most prominent medical supporters of state laws to mandate health insurance, and later of the CCMC majority, and of their political heirs.

Hugh Cabot and Ernest Boas exemplified this point of view. Hugh Cabot, a cousin of Richard, eagerly promoted reorganizing medical care into hierarchies dominated by academics. "The individual physician," Cabot insisted, "is no longer in a position to come to safe judgments without conferring with his colleagues."[73]

Ernest Boas, medical director of Montefiore Hospital in New York City and a pioneer in the treatment of chronic illness, deplored the incompetence of most doctors outside academic medicine. Cabot convicted the profession of ignorance; Boas disparaged scientific pretensions as well. Young doctors, he complained, suffered from the misguided conviction that every procedure must have a causal mechanism established by science.[74]

These convictions were shared by a small but increasing number of doctors who had access to the press, foundation executives, and liberal political leaders. Roger I. Lee, for example, had devised a formula for building and distributing hospitals by assuming that good medical care was what the leaders of the medical profession practiced and taught.[75] The doctors who shared this assumption used it to propose reorganizing other aspects of medical care.

In the late 1930s, faculty members at a few leading medical schools, notably Harvard, Johns Hopkins, and Yale, tested a new political strategy. They tried to organize a coalition for new health policy that consisted entirely of doctors and to advertise their views to the general public as sound medical advice.

This new strategy was used in 1937, in a two-volume survey titled *American Medicine: Expert Testimony Out of Court*. The testimony consisted of excerpts from letters about health policy and the organization of practice from 2,100 doctors. The letters were solicited by an organization called the American Foundation, which was led by a journalist, Esther Everett Lape, who was a political ally of Eleanor Roosevelt. The doctors who wrote letters defied the silence imposed by professional etiquette about conflict within the medical

[73] Hugh Cabot, *The Patient's Dilemma* (New York: Reynal and Hitchcock, 1940), 1-2, 39-40, 81-82, 214. Hugh Cabot to Michael M. Davis, April 19, 1939, Davis Papers.

[74] Ernest P. Boas, *The Unseen Plague: Chronic Disease* (New York: J. J. Augustin, 1940), 19-21.

[75] Lee and Jones, *The Fundamentals*, 6.

profession. After Lape prepared a digest of the book for the *New York Times*, other newspapers and magazines publicized its contents.[76]

Expert Testimony was followed by a manifesto sponsored by fourteen academic physicians. They demanded a national health policy that would subsidize medical education, biomedical research, constructing hospitals and laboratories, and the medical expenses of the indigent. This policy, they said, should be administered by voluntary agencies, and by local, state, and federal government. The authors of the CCMC majority report had advocated regional hierarchies of doctors and institutions as a strategy to improve the accountability and therefore the quality of practice. The authors of the manifesto made the same proposal more diplomatically, declaring vaguely that public funds should be spent to raise the standards of medical practice.[77]

The authors of the manifesto were, however, as firmly committed as the CCMC majority to hierarchy in medical organization. The members of what soon became a larger organization supporting the manifesto, the Committee of 430, were all specialists with prestigious institutional affiliations: senior faculty members and chiefs of services at major medical schools and teaching hospitals; officers of major associations of specialists; biomedical scientists, including a Nobel laureate; deans of medical schools; and prominent public health leaders, notably the surgeon general of the United States. Each of them was listed with his or her affiliation to make plain their distinction.[78] Many of the signers were eager to provoke conflict within the profession. For instance, James Howard Means, the Jackson Professor of Clinical Medicine at Harvard, serving in 1938 as president of the American College of Physicians, scandalized his colleagues by promoting the manifesto at their annual meeting.[79]

This medical intellectual elite believed that doctors should set health policy. For example, John P. Peters, Ely Professor of Medicine at Yale and secretary of the Committee of 430, assumed that what he called the productive services of medicine were controlled

[76] Rorty, *American Medicine Mobilizes* 82ff; Burrow, *AMA*, 201; James Howard Means, *Doctors, People and Government* (Boston: Little, Brown and Co., 1953), 143-147; Julius Richmond, *Currents in American Medicine* (Cambridge: Harvard University Press, 1969), 16.

[77] "The Committee of Physicians for the Presentation of Certain Principles and Proposals on the Provision of Medical Care." *New England Journal of Medicine*, November 11, 1937, 217: 798-800.

[78] *Ibid.*, 800.

[79] Piersol, *Gateway of Honor*, 146.

by doctors who practiced at educational and research institutes and their hospitals. Other doctors, he said, had "fallen almost completely into the derivative position of distributor or dispenser."[80]

Despite their exclusion from the Committee of 430, the lay reformers who regarded themselves as members of a vanguard believed that in 1938 they were once again on the verge of victory. They held a National Health Conference that summer to celebrate the strategy that had guided campaigns to reform medical care since the American Association for Labor Legislation was organized early in the century. The conference was convened by Josephine Roche, assistant secretary of the Treasury, who chaired an Interdepartmental Committee to Coordinate Health and Welfare. This committee was preparing to send President Roosevelt a proposal for a National Health Program: Federal grants to states to subsidize maternal and child services and compulsory insurance programs, and direct federal payments to support the temporarily disabled, the blind, and crippled children, and a national hospital construction program. The committee also reaffirmed the recommendations of the majority of the CCMC for reorganizing health services. The conference, called to endorse the committee's report, was attended by two hundred leaders from the health professions, hospital associations, state and local government, labor unions, and farmers' and women's organizations.[81]

---

[80] Rorty, *American Medicine Mobilizes*, 93-94. *Cf.* "The Committee," 798; John Fulton, *Harvey Cushing* (Springfield, Ill.: Charles C. Thomas, 1946), 650. The new strategy of the medical elite did not appeal to Surgeon General Parran. Although he eventually signed the committee's manifesto, he wrote Josephine Roche, assistant secretary of the Treasury, that the document was "a very weak and unsatisfactory statement." He made clear that he had not participated in writing the document. Parran would remain loyal to the vanguard of reform until the war. (Rarran to Roche, April 16, 1937, Mary Switzer Papers, Box 3, Folder 32, Schlesinger Library, Radcliffe College.)

[81] *Report and Recommendations on National Health by the Interdepartmental Committee to Coordinate Health and Welfare Activities.* In *Health Security: Message From the President of the United States*, U.S. Congress, House, 76th Congress, 1st Session, Document no. 120, 3ff.; The Technical Committee on Medical Care, Interdepartmental Committee to Coordinate Health and Welfare Activities, *The Need for a National Health Program* (Washington, D.C., USGPO, 1938); *cf.* Rorty, *American Medicine Mobilizes*, 43, "the Committee's report reaffirms the 'medical center' idea expressed in 1932 by the majority report of the CCMC." Rorty's statement (p.16), "the National Health Conference had the effect of changing almost overnight the whole alignment of forces" began the myth of the Conference. Josephine Roche's enthusiasm is widely reported in secondary sources; what she actually wrote to the president in her letter transmitting the report (Roche to Franklin D. Roosevelt, January 12, 1939, *Report and Recommendations*, 3) was, "The interdepartmental committee believes that the findings and

The conference was a euphoric experience for the members of the vanguard. In the keynote address, Michael Davis eulogized them and attacked the AMA. Health reform, he told the conference, would now move into the public eye. After the conference, the lay reformers took a poll among themselves about when the new program would be enacted.[82] Louis Reed later recalled that half of them believed the National Health Program would become law in 1939; the others predicted a delay of up to four years.[83]

The vanguard assumed that agreement about symbolic issues was a sufficient basis for a political coalition. They were confident that participants in a conference who agreed about the achievements of men in white and who declared, according to the proceedings, that death took most of its holiday from the first year of childhood to the early years of adult life would also agree on the substance of legislation.[84]

These dramatic phrases in the proceedings suggest a consensus about policy that did not exist. Several of the prominent doctors who attended the conference emphasized the lack of consensus by dissociating themselves from the National Health Program. S. S. Goldwater, former director of Mt. Sinai Hospital in New York City and a member of the committee that had drafted the model health insurance bill in 1916, insisted that medical care was not the most immediate problem for the American people. John P. Peters, speaking on behalf of the Committee of 430, agreed with him. Alice Hamilton, pioneer in industrial medicine, the first woman faculty member at Harvard, and an advocate of medical care reform for thirty years, accused the Interdepartmental Committee of confusing health and economic problems.[85]

These doctors exhibited a new political strategy. For two decades, a vanguard of lay reformers and their medical allies had pressed forward without calculating the political feasibility of their goals. Now,

---

proposals of the technical report . . . are amply corroborated by professional and lay experience and opinion." Cf. Hirshfield, *The Lost Reform*, 104-108, and Monte M. Poen, *Harry S. Truman Versus the Medical Lobby: The Genesis of Medicare* (Columbia: University of Missouri Press, 1979).

[82] *The Nation's Health*. Discussions at the National Health Conference, July 18, 19, 20, 1938, Washington, D.C. Called by the Interdepartmental Committee to Coordinate Health and Welfare Activities (Washington, D.C.: USGPO, 1939), 102-103.

[83] Hirshfield, *The Lost Reform*, 108, 209. The poll was taken at a party attended by, among others, I. S. Falk, Margaret Klem, Joseph Mountin, George St. John Perrot, Louis Reed, and Nathan Sinai.

[84] See above, Notes 4, 5, 8.

[85] *The Nation's Health*, 58, 61-62, 60.

prominent doctors with deep roots in the reform movement, acknowledged that most Americans accorded low priority to changes in the way medical care was organized and financed. Like the members of the vanguard, Goldwater, Hamilton, and Peters wanted health to have higher priority in American politics. Unlike the vanguard, however, they urged gradualism and accommodation as alternatives to advocacy of comprehensive reform.

The vanguard, led by Surgeon General Thomas Parran and Arthur Altmeyer, chairman of the Social Security Board, was, however, in charge of advocating new health policy within the federal government. Parran was the principal spokesman for the Administration on medical care. He owed his position to prominent lay reformers. Governor Franklin Roosevelt had appointed him health commissioner of New York at the suggestion of Edgar Sydenstriker and John Kingsbury of the Milbank Memorial Fund. Parran seemed to have no doubts about the assumptions of the vanguard, even though he had signed the manifesto of the Committee of 430. As he told the National Health Conference, medicine and public health should lead economics.[86]

The National Health Program was doomed, despite the euphoria of its proponents. President Roosevelt transmitted the program to Congress for careful study rather than for action.[87] Senator Robert F. Wagner introduced a bill to implement the program, which his staff had drafted with assistance from employees of the Social Security Board and the Public Health Service, but it was accorded low priority by labor unions and farm organizations. The president then announced that he supported only those sections of the bill calling for federal assistance to build hospitals.[88]

Despite such weak support for their program, Parran, Altmeyer, and their staffs rejected a compromise offered by the American

[86] Furman, *A Profile*, 393-394. In the mid 1930s, Parran made such abrasive pronouncements as, "The medical profession is increasingly unable to provide for all the people the minimum essentials of medical care" (1937) and "the health service of tomorrow inevitably will conform to the governmental framework" (1934).

[87] *Report and Recommendations . . . Health Security Message . . .*, p. 2. After saying he recommended only "careful study," President Roosevelt inverted the priorities of the medical care reformers: "The essence of the program recommended by the Committee is Federal-State cooperation."

[88] Witte, *Social Security Perspectives*, 333-334; cf. Frederick D. Mott and Milton I. Roemer, *Rural Health and Medical Care* (New York: McGraw-Hill Book Co., 1948), 468. Only the Farmers' Union consistently supported compulsory insurance. The Farm Bureau and the Grange were willing to support only hospital construction and public health extension. For a different interpretation of the failure of reform in the late 1930s see Starr, *Social Transformation of American Medicine*, 275-279.

Medical Association and the American Hospital Association. A few months after the National Health Conference, the AMA House of Delegates, in an emergency meeting, had voted to support the proposed National Health Program with the exception of grants to the states to subsidize mandatory insurance. Shortly thereafter, the AMA and the AHA had jointly endorsed federal subsidy for hospital construction under local control coupled with the expansion of voluntary health insurance.[89]

Parran and Altmeyer refused to accept this compromise. In 1940, during Senate hearings on the bill to subsidize the construction of hospitals, for instance, Parran asserted that the federal government must regulate the quality of medical care because most doctors and community leaders were not competent to operate hospitals properly.[90]

Parran was, however, treated gently by representatives of the interest groups whose offers of compromise he scorned. Senator Robert Taft, a defender of the rights of voluntary hospitals and the states, politely admonished him for insensitivity to state and local responsibilities. The president of the American Hospital Association suggested that the Public Health Service lacked expertise to regulate hospitals. Morris Fishbein praised the use of relief funds to construct hospitals in the worst years of the Depression and endorsed the goals of the Administration's hospital bill but suggested, in mild phrases, that the federal government need not regulate hospitals. To organized medicine and the hospital industry, obtaining subsidies was, for the first time, more important than annihilating doctrinal enemies.[91]

Nevertheless, the hospital bill, like the rest of the National Health

[89] Burrow, *AMA*, 217-221, 246. The AMA leaders met privately with the Interdepartmental Committee and offered to support the entire program except for encouragement of the States to mount compulsory insurance programs, according to Arthur Altmeyer, then one of three members of the Social Security Board, in *The Formative Years of Social Security* (Madison: University of Wisconsin Press, 1966), 96. *Cf.* Hirshfield, *The Lost Reform*, 124-125, for a different interpretation. Michael Davis wrote to I. S. Falk on February 16, 1939 (Davis Papers, M-1), to express his anger and surprise that the AMA and the hospital associations were making an alliance. Poen, *Harry S. Truman*, 26, arrayed many of the same data but reaches a different conclusion.

[90] *Construction of Hospitals*, Hearings before a subcommittee of the Committee on Education and Labor, U.S. Senate, 76th Congress, 2nd Session, S. 3230, March 18-19, 1940, *passim; cf.* "The Wagner-George-Lea Bill . . . ," *Journal of the American Medical Association*, April 13, 1940, 114: 1365.

[91] *Construction of Hospitals, passim.*

Program, was not enacted. The bill passed the Senate in 1940 but did not come to a vote in the House as a result, its supporters said, of other pressing business. The lack of strong commitment to the bill by the president most likely encouraged opposition among congressmen who were not eager to mediate conflicts between interest groups in their districts who wanted subsidies and federal officials who wanted to control what doctors did in community hospitals.[92]

The defeat of the hospital bill taught different political lessons to the groups advocating new health policy. Most of the lay reformers in the vanguard and a few of their medical allies decided that, in the future, they should not support permissive legislation.[93] The primacy of medical care in social policy must never again be compromised. Henceforth they would seek a whole loaf, having failed to get half of one.

Advocates of federal subsidy within academic medicine, the hospital associations, and the Public Health Service reached a different conclusion. They decided to mobilize the enthusiasm of the public and its elected representatives for medical science on behalf of policy to increase the supply of medical services—of hospitals, of biomedical research and, eventually, of doctors.[94] They would separate the problems of how much care was available and how it was organized from the troublesome, polarizing issue of how individuals paid for care.

[92] Altmeyer, *The Formative Years*, 126; Hirshfield, *The Lost Reform*, 157-158; J. Joseph Hutmacher, *Senator Robert K. Wagner and the Rise of Urban Liberalism* (New York: Atheneum, 1968), 266-267; Poen, *Harry S. Truman*, 26-27.

[93] Hirshfield, *The Lost Reform*, 164.

[94] Mobilization on behalf of policy for research has been addressed by Stephen P. Strickland, *Politics, Science, and Dread Disease* (Cambridge: Harvard University Press, 1972).

VI

The Second World War and Health
Policy: Britain, 1939-1945

BY THE LATE 1930s, although individuals and interest groups in Britain disagreed about how to define and govern regions, there was no controversy about the desirability of creating hierarchies of hospitals coordinated with other services. Moreover, unlike the United States, where prominent doctors had begun to separate the issue of increasing the supply of health services from general social policy, British interest groups continued to emphasize the social as well as the scientific justification for national health policy.

Advocates of hierarchical regionalism within the Ministry of Health became more aggressive. In 1936, Sir Arthur McNalty, Newman's successor as chief medical officer, doubted whether the public would accept local authorities as administrators of specialist services for the whole community that were based upon hospitals. A year later, however, he endorsed proposals to promote coordination by local authorities of voluntary hospitals and general practitioners.[1] By 1938, civil servants were encouraging the ministry's advisory committee to recommend that they press local authorities to cooperate with voluntary hospitals through joint boards. Later that year, senior civil servants agreed that the ministry should promote comprehensive regional plans to coordinate health services, including specialized medical care, which should no longer be conceived as simply an additional insurance benefit.[2]

TOWARD A POSTWAR HOSPITAL POLICY

As the threat of war grew, the consensus about how hospitals should be organized became the basis for civil defense policy. In

---

[1] "Memorandum on Provision of Specialist Services by the C.M.O.," MH 80/24, PRO. (A memo of March 15, 1937, reporting a meeting of December 10, 1936.)

[2] The material quoted here is in MH 80/24-30, PRO; *cf.* John E. Pater, *The Making of the National Health Service* (London: King Edward's Fund, 1981); *cf.* Sir Arthur S. MacNalty, "Medicine and the Public Health," *British Medical Journal*, July 3, 1948, ii: 6-9.

June 1938, the ministry created an Emergency Hospital Service. Within newly established regions, public and voluntary hospitals were graded and coordinated by staff of the ministry. Consultants were paid full-time salaries and were distributed among these regions.[3]

During the next seven years, the Emergency Hospital Service, its name gradually changing to Emergency Medical Service, became a national hospital service. The ministry set performance standards for medical and administrative services, established regional networks of diagnostic and treatment centers and of consultants, organized a national blood transfusion program, introduced uniform pay scales for professional and lay staff, and constructed or renovated facilities that provided 80,000 new hospital beds.[4] As a result of the EMS, the minister told a meeting of a committee of the War Cabinet in 1941, Britain now had, for the first time in its history, enough hospitals to meet the needs of the entire population.[5]

By September 1939, the civil servants were planning a national hospital system to be implemented after the war. Sir Arthur McNalty now believed that national ownership of hospitals was inevitable because the country would become accustomed to the state controlling them during the war. The medical profession would, he asserted, prefer nationalizing hospitals to having them controlled by local authorities.[6] A deputy secretary proposed to create a national hospital system by making financial assistance to the voluntary hospitals contingent upon their either grouping themselves into regional councils or forming joint organizations with local authorities.[7]

The implications of the wartime reorganization of hospitals for postwar policy were also discussed outside the ministry. A com-

---

[3] C. L. Dunn, *The Emergency Medical Services*, vol. I (London: HMSO, 1952), *passim*; *The Times* said on April 6, 1939, that Ministry of Health staff were to be "partly regionalized . . . for the provision of medical services to meet a possible national emergency."

[4] Dunn, *Emergency*; Richard M. Titmuss, *Problems of Social Policy* (London: HMSO and Longman's Green, 1950), 502.

[5] War Cabinet, Lord President's Committee, October 15, 1941, MH 80/34, PRO.

[6] A. MacNalty to E. J. Maude, "Proposed National Hospital Services," September 21, 1939, MH 80/24, PRO.

[7] A. N. Rucker to E. J. Maude, September 29, 1939, "Proposed National Hospital Service," MH 80/24, PRO. Sir Edward Forber, "Regional Organization of Hospital Services," traced the growing consensus on the issue since the Dawson Report. Another document, "Summary of Recommendations of Certain Bodies," arrayed other data in favor of hierarchical regionalism.

mittee of the British Hospitals Association asserted in December 1939 that voluntary hospitals should be coordinated within a national health service.[8] The authors of a paper issued by Political and Economic Planning, the centrist study group, suggested that the Emergency Hospital Service become a permanent National Service led by regional officers appointed by the Ministry of Health.[9] In 1939, the authors of a Labour party pamphlet, *War and the Medical Services*, proposed that local authorities rather than the central government coordinate health services on a regional basis.[10]

The Minister of Health encouraged the Nuffield Provincial Hospitals Trust, which was established in 1939 to advocate regional coordination of voluntary hospitals, to stimulate public discussion of postwar hospital policy. In an exchange of letters that they released to the press in mid-January 1941, the minister and the chairman of the Trust agreed that postwar policy for hospitals was of major importance. The minister endorsed the Trust's belief that hospital planning should occur for regions that were larger than existing local government jurisdictions.[11] The chairman of the Trust's Medical Advisory Committee reported in the *Lancet* two weeks later that the minister agreed with him that some form of regional hospital organization would be necessary after the war.[12]

During the next ten months, officials of the ministry devised policy for postwar hospital services. They assumed that reverting to prewar conditions would be impossible.[13] The officials quickly agreed, moreover, that adequate hospital facilities should be available for the whole population. These facilities should, moreover, be planned and coordinated in regions that were substantially larger than existing local government areas. In each region one or more hospitals should be attached to a medical school.[14] The civil servants

[8] BHA, Provisional Central Council, 5 December 1939. British Hospitals Contributory Schemes Papers, LSE.

[9] PEP cited in Pater, *Making of the National Health Service*, 19.

[10] *War and the Medical Services* (London: Labour Research Department, 1939). This and other pamphlets are collected in Medical Planning Commission, 1941-42, vol. 1075, BMA Registry.

[11] The letters were released to the press on January 15, 1941. A *Times* leader, "A New Hospital Service," traced the regional idea from the Dawson Report to the present. Letters and clippings in MH 77/25, PRO.

[12] Sir E. Farquhar Buzzard, "Post War Hospital Policy," *The Lancet*, February 1, 1941, i: 155-156.

[13] Pater, *Making of the National Health Service*, 21, paraphrasing a document he noted in MH 77/26. It may be what Maude believed and said privately, but it is a stronger statement than what he wrote at the time.

[14] "Office Committee on Past War Hospital Policy," January 24, 1941, MH 77/22, PRO.

were divided, however, about the authority of local officials. Some senior officials believed that hospitals should be managed by regional bodies that were independent of local government. Others emphasized the ministry's long-standing alliance with local authorities.[15]

The scope of planning for postwar policy rapidly expanded. The new chief medical officer, Sir Wilson Jameson, who had succeeded McNalty in 1940, told representatives of the Nuffield Trust in February 1941 that all medical services must be regionalized. But his colleagues urged him to be more cautious. Editing the minutes of this meeting, Jameson changed the words "must" to "might have to be" and "all" to "other."[16] The limits of consensus had not yet been tested.

The Nuffield Trust, exploiting its access to the ministry, antagonized many local officials by holding public meetings at which its representatives tried to persuade local authorities and voluntary hospitals to establish regional councils.[17] Some local officials began to suspect the Trust of plotting, as Charles (later Lord) Latham, a leader of the London County Council said, to steal the people's municipal hospitals.[18]

Not everyone in local government shared these concerns. A few months before Latham's attack, W. Allen Daley, MOH of London, writing unofficially to a friend in the ministry, endorsed regional coordination of voluntary and public hospitals. Moreover, he said that he approved of maintaining the independence of teaching hospitals if public hospitals in London were also treated as a special case. Many local authorities, he continued, were too small to administer an adequate hospital service. Daley's commitment to reorganizing hospital services was stronger than his loyalty to his political masters. Unlike prominent LCC councillors, he complained, he was willing to sacrifice local control. The most difficult problem, Daley concluded, was how to use hospitals efficiently, not, as Somerville

[15] For example, "Notes by Mr. Rucker," 6 February 1941; H. S. de Montmorency to E. J. Maude, February 12, 1941, MH 77/22, PRO.

[16] "Hospital Regionalization," 6 February 1941 (quoting Jameson, with corrections in his hand), MH 80/24, PRO.

[17] Memorandum by Minister of Health to War Cabinet. Lord President's Committee on Post War Hospital Policy, October 14, 1941, included a chronology of events. The chronology stated that "disquietude" in "local government circles" came to the minister's attention in August 1941. MH 77/22, PRO. Cf. Pater, Making of the National Health Service.

[18] Charles Latham, "The Case for Public Control," The Star, August 12, 1941, 2. Clipping in MH 77/25, PRO. In the same article, however, Latham defended the hierarchical regional organization of services "with one national standard."

Hastings and other leaders of the LCC argued, how to create a comprehensive state medical service.[19]

The Cabinet authorized Minister of Health Ernest Brown to announce a policy for a postwar hospital service in order to allay what Brown called the disquietude of local officials. In response to a Parliamentary Question on October 9, 1941, he declared that the Government intended to ensure that, after the war, a comprehensive hospital service would make appropriate treatment readily available to every person in need of it. This service, Brown emphasized, would be administered by local authorities collaborating with voluntary hospitals. The work of hospitals should, however, be coordinated in areas which were substantially larger than counties or county boroughs. Replying to questions about policy for establishing a comprehensive national health service, Brown insisted that the hospital service must be considered first.[20]

The alliance between the ministry and the Nuffield Trust continued despite Brown's statement that the Government was committed to a postwar hospital service controlled by local authorities. Before Brown announced this commitment, the ministry and the Trust had agreed to cosponsor regional surveys of hospital facilities. The Trust was so deeply involved in discussions about postwar hospital policy that its chairman confided to Sir Wilson Jameson that he had given the *Times* two weeks advance notice of the statement the minister would make to Parliament. He seemed to believe that the Trust alone had received advance information, which, in fact, the ministry had shared with seven other interest groups.[21]

In early 1942, leaders of two of these groups complained to the ministry that the Trust had too much influence. The County Councils Association and the Association of Municipal Corporations criticized the boundaries of the regions assigned to the surveyors chosen jointly by the Trust and the ministry. But the associations, themselves committed to regionalization and hierarchy, were will-

[19] W. Allen Daley to A. N. Rucker, March 4, 1941, MH 77/22, PRO.

[20] Hansard, *Parliamentary Debates*, House of Commons, 5th Ser. vol. 374, October 9, 1941, cols. 1116-1120; Instructions to Minister for Parliament, October 9, 1941, MH 77/22, PRO.

[21] William Goodenough to Wilson Jameson, 35, September, 1941, MH 77/25, PRO. On other interest groups see Pater, *Making of the National Health Service*, 29-31. The same month the Nuffield Provincial Hospitals Trust published *A National Hospital Service: A Memorandum on the Coordination of Hospital Service* (Oxford: The Trust, 1941), which was timed to coincide with the government's announcement of policy. This pamphlet called for the division of the country into hospital regions, and the formation of a Voluntary Hospital Central Council in each region.

ing to compromise. Despite their hostility to the Trust and voluntary hospitals, the representatives of the associations agreed that surveyors could explore neighboring areas without defining explicit regional boundaries.[22] Within a few months, however, efforts by representatives of the Trust to organize ad hoc regional councils and their demand for early publication and local dicussion of the surveys created more antagonism than the ministry could afford to ignore. Sir John Maude, the permanent secretary, told the chairman of the Trust that the Government was not committed to any particular form of regional organization to manage hospitals after the war. The ministry would, moreover, publish the results of the surveys on its own schedule.[23]

The surveyors based their judgments on implicit standards for the quantity and quality of hospital services. Each of the teams assumed that the organization of hospitals into hierarchies was desirable. Only one team, the surveyors for the Northeastern Area, refused to adopt a quantitative standard for how many beds were needed. The other nine teams proposed ideal bed-to-population ratios of between 2.5 and 5:1000, either before or after arraying their data.[24]

Officials of the ministry were not interested in establishing uniform ratios. They did not discuss using standard bed-to-population ratios at the first meeting of surveying officers in October 1942.[25] The civil servant who coordinated the surveys believed that it was impossible to set ideal standards of hospital accommodation. In the same memorandum, however, he alluded to standards proposed before the war by the Society of Medical Officers of Health and to

[22] Minutes of a Conference: E. J. Maude, W. Jameson, Nuffield Trust, County Councils Association and Association of Municipal Corporations. January 28, 1942, MH 77/26, PRO.

[23] Minutes of a Meeting between E. J. Maude and W. M. Goodenough (Nuffield Trust), March 12, 1942, MH 77/19, PRO. A chronological file of pertinent documents in the formation of hospital policy is in MH 80/34, PRO.

[24] Ministry of Health, *Hospital Survey*, 10 vols. (London: HMSO, 1945 and 1946). The exception is vol. 5, 13. Most of the others used ratios of 4 or 5:1000; but one used 2.5 and one 3.5:1000. One was silent. *Cf.* R. S. Aitken *et al., Scottish Hospitals Survey: General Introduction to the Reports* (Edinburg, HMSO, 1949), 11, where a ratio of 8:1000 was recommended for acute general beds in "closely knit industrial areas." Moreover, the "hospital surveyors in all regions had been unanimous about the need for a regional organization. . . ." *Cf.* Sir George Godber, "Regional Devolution and the National Health Service," in Edward Crafen, ed., *Regional Devolution and Social Policy* (London: Macmillan, 1975), 60ff.

[25] [English] *Hospital Survey*, vol. 6, 16, (written by George Godber); the Minutes of the Meeting of Surveying Officers, October 5, 1942, MH 77/19, PRO.

those used by the United States Public Health Service.[26] Before the surveys were published, moreover, a senior official of the ministry discussed planning standards with American officials and foundation executives.[27] Unlike the Americans, who rationalized their subjective assessments, even presenting them as an equation, the British simply deferred to expert opinion, even though this meant that each survey team used different standards. Like their American contemporaries, however, most of the British surveyors used a standard of between four and five acute general hospital beds per thousand population. Moreover, like American experts, they assumed that an increase in the quantity of beds was the best remedy for deficient quality.

The results of the surveys reinforced the agreement between the ministry and medical interest groups about the substance of postwar policy. Though not officially published until 1945, the results were widely distributed in draft and were endorsed by every faction in medical and general politics. The surveyors agreed on the need to create regions that transcended the boundaries of local authorities, to redistribute consultants from the large cities, to limit the surgery performed in cottage or general practitioner hospitals, and to reorganize services for the chronically ill.[28] Each of these issues was controversial when the surveys began. By 1945, the ministry regarded agreement among the surveyors as further justification of Government policy. The surveys, a civil servant wrote in 1946, had documented the awkwardness and inefficiency of existing hospital services.[29]

SUBORDINATING CONTROVERSY

Support for the postwar hospital policy announced in 1940 grew between 1941 and 1943. Leaders of the general practitioners, consultants, and medical officers of health reasserted their commitment to organizing hospital and specialist services in regional hierarchies.

[26] N. F. McNicoll to Stephen Taylor, June 3, 1943, MH 77/20, PRO; "Cost of Hospitals and other Institutions," Memorandum Submitted to the Ministry of Health, Departmental Committee, by the Society of Medical Officers of Health, July 1934. Reprinted from Public Health, in SMOH Papers, E-5. Wellcome Unit, Oxford.

[27] C. T. Maitland, "Hospitals in the United States," The Lancet, January 24, 1948, i: 152-154; January 31, 1948, i: 186-188.

[28] M. F. McNichol to W. Jameson, April 13, 1944, MH 77/24, PRO.

[29] J. Pater to E. J. Maude, May 5, 1946, on the occasion of the Nuffield Trust's issuing a summary of the surveys, The Hospital Surveys: The Domesday Book of the Hospital Service, MH 77/25, PRO.

They consistently subordinated intense conflicts within the profession to their fundamental agreement about the organization of services. Under the influence of war, moreover, each political party made a commitment to establishing a postwar health service to provide comprehensive care to almost everyone in Britain.[30]

A Medical Planning Commission, organized by the BMA in 1941 to resolve conflict within the profession, issued an interim report in 1942 urging the grouping of hospitals in hierarchies as a prerequisite to making all necessary services available to everyone.[31] At the first meeting of the MPC, Lord Dawson declared that regionalizing hospitals and health services was the most important question to settle. Sir Frederick Menzies, the former chief medical officer of the LCC, supported Dawson's belief that priority should be accorded to the organization rather than the substance or the results of medical care.[32]

A month before the Government announced that it was committed to a postwar hospital policy, the MPC's Hospital Committee approved a recommendation to regionalize both hospital and doctor services. Participants in this discussion included Lord Dawson; Allen Daley; Sir Farquhar Buzzard, Regius Professor of Medicine at Oxford and chairman of the Nuffield Trust's Medical Advisory Committee; Somerville Hastings; Lord Moran, who was president of the Royal College of Physicians, Prime Minister Churchill's physician, and a former medical school dean; and Sir Weldon Dalrymple-Champnys, deputy to Sir Wilson Jameson. Daley and Hastings addressed the hostility of general practitioners to municipal government by suggesting that medical issues, rather than the boundaries of counties or boroughs, should determine the size and shape of regions. A region, the other committee members agreed, should be a large area within which all hospital services were coordinated.[33]

[30] Frank Honigsbaum, *The Division in British Medicine* (New York: St. Martin's 1979), 189.

[31] Medical Planning Commission, *Draft Interim Report* (London: British Medical Association, 1942), 5, 14.

[32] Dawson and Menzies are quoted in Sir Frederick Menzies, "Regionalization of Hospitals and Health Services," *British Medical Journal*, July 12, 1941, ii: 60-61. *Cf.* "Notes" for discussion, July 16, 1941, Medical Planning Commission, Hospitals Committee, vol. 2075, BMA Registry.

[33] The betrayal of Local Authorities by their leading defenders in medicine was prefaced by a second position paper on regionalization, made available at the committee meeting of September 4, 1941, which extended the concept from hospitals to medical services as a whole. Hospitals Committee Minutes, September 4, 1941, vol. 2075, BMA Registry.

Two months later, Dalrymple-Champnys assured the MPC committee that maintaining support for hierarchical regionalization within the medical profession was more important to the ministry than its public assurances to local authorities. The minister had promised Parliament that local authorities would be responsible for the postwar hospital service. His emissary contradicted him, telling the committee that the minister had no position on the structure and jurisdiction of regional councils and that he preferred to let the matter remain as fluid as possible.[34] The civil servant's priority, as Jameson commented a short time later, was to maintain agreement among doctors that their continued isolation from each other was in the interests neither of themselves nor of the public.[35]

Although the MPC's interim report was tabled by the BMA's representative body, most doctors agreed with its priorities for reorganizing hospital and medical services after the war. Most GPs, BMA's opinion polls revealed, wanted hospital care to be paid for by the central government and rendered in institutions managed by regional boards independent of local authorities. The report was tabled mainly because of its recommendation that general practitioners be paid full-time salaries. Moreover, many BMA members preferred a postwar health service that would be managed by a national corporation rather than by the ministry, as the MPC recommended. This corporation would, however, establish regional councils composed of representatives of local authorities, voluntary hospitals, and doctors. During the discussion of the interim report at a BMA meeting, a few general practitioners worried that, as a result of medical school control of hospital hierarchies, they might be excluded completely from hospital practice.[36]

A few months later a group called Medical Planning Research, consisting of two hundred doctors under the age of forty-five, endorsed regional hierarchies in the context of wider social reforms. Like abolishing poverty and redistributing wealth, they argued, reorganizing medical care was a postwar obligation. A medical service based on what they called key hospitals should be available to everyone. The cost of medical care was a trivial issue, the group

<hr />

[34] Minutes, Hospitals Committee, November 18, 1941, vol. 2075, BMA Registry. Honigsbaum reported, without a source (185), that Wilson Jameson worked hard to influence the recommendations of the MPC. It is thus not clear whether or not his deputy exceeded his instructions.

[35] Honigsbaum, *The Division*, 185.

[36] BMA, Annual Representative Meeting, "Medical Planning Commission," *British Medical Journal Supplement*, September 1, 26, October 10, 1942, ii: *passim*.

said, provided that it did not encroach on other social priorities.[37]

Another group, the doctors who spoke for the Fabian Society and the Socialist Medical Association, also gave priority to creating hierarchical medical services in regions. In 1940, Somerville Hastings, in a Fabian pamphlet, declared that the largest possible number of hospitals should be grouped together and administered as single units.[38] The Fabians also asserted that the first requirement for a healthy nation was that doctors acquire current medical knowledge by participating in regional networks.[39] According to David Stark Murray of the SMA, achieving optimum health required both coordinating services in regional hierarchies and more investment in medical research.[40] Hastings and Stark Murray agreed that the advantages of modern medical science could be diffused best by changing the organization of medical care.[41]

Henry Cohen, then professor of medicine at Liverpool, emphasized the consensus about postwar medical policy among doctors in a paper written late in 1942 and circulated by the BMA as a pamphlet early the next year. According to Cohen, measures to improve the general welfare and regionalized medical care were both necessary to achieve the highest possible standard of positive health. Doctors lacked expert knowledge of the cure for want, ignorance, and squalor. Laymen were, however, unable to understand the po-

---

[37] Medical Planning Research, "Interim General Report," *The Lancet Supplement*, November 21, 1942, ii: 599-622, *passim*.

[38] Somerville Hastings, *The Hospital Services: A Policy for the War and Post War Period* (London: Victor Gollancz for the Fabian Society, December 1941), 8. Hastings had chosen solidarity with his medical rather than with his socialist colleagues two months earlier in the MPC Hospitals Committee saying, "no lay authority can ever be permitted to interfere in medical matters" (16).

[39] Joan Simeon Clarke, "National Health Insurance," in William A. Robson, ed., *Social Society* (London: Published for the Fabian Society by George Allen and Unwin, 1943). She called explicitly for hierarchical "teamwork" (90).

[40] D. Stark Murray, "National Medical Service," in *ibid.*, 395-403.

[41] D. Stark Murray, *Health for All* (London: Victor Gollancz, 1942), 7, 45. The interpretation of the SMA given here differs from D. Stark Murray's in *Why a National Health Service: the Part Played by the Socialist Medical Association* (London: Pemberton Books, 1971).

The consensus on postwar medical care policy within the profession was publicized outside the profession. The Liberal party endorsed regionalization by the federation of local authorities and urged that the "unit of the Health Service should be a local health centre." The Labour party compartmentalized general social reform and medical care. Labour also urged a full-time salaried medical service organized by a "comprehensive plan" of regional hospitals. *Health for the People* (London: Liberal Publications Department, 1942); *National Service for Health* (London: The Labour Party, April 1943), 2-3, 6.

tentialities of the health services. Therefore doctors should acknowledge the importance of general social policy but let laymen design and implement it. The public and politicians should let doctors and officials responsive to them allocate resources to medical care. If this bargain could be struck, Cohen concluded, the medical profession would embrace a postwar policy that included universal entitlement, free choice of physician, hospitals regionalized beyond the effective control of local government, and financial security for general practitioners.[42]

William Beveridge's report, *Social Insurance and Allied Services*, published at the end of 1942, summarized and strengthened the consensus within the medical profession about postwar policy for medical care. Beveridge was a leading Liberal intellectual, who had been an official of the Treasury and the director of the London School of Economics. He had been appointed in 1941 by the War Cabinet to chair a committee on postwar social policy. Beveridge dominated the committee. The report was a personal document, signed only by him, which received considerable publicity because of the public hearings that preceded it and the attractiveness of its proposals for comprehensive social security and health policy after the war.

According to Beveridge, the goal of health policy was the attainment of positive health. Achieving this goal should, he said, take precedence over other uses of public and personal resources. Restoring sick people to health, he insisted, was a duty of the state, in cooperation with the sick themselves. A sick person's duty was, however, mainly to comply with medical advice, since the Ministry of Health should provide, without any conditions, whatever medical treatment each person required. Medical care, he asserted, should be comprehensive and free, and should be provided as the absolute first priority of public policy.[43]

Beveridge was inconsistent about health policy. On the one hand, he wanted the state to establish a free, comprehensive health service. On the other, he repeatedly declared that he wanted the state to guarantee citizens' entitlement to what he called basic doctor and hospital services that would be paid for by compulsory insurance. Moreover, he believed that services paid for by insurance

---

[42] Henry Cohen, "A Comprehensive Health Service," reprinted from *Agenda*, February 1943, in the BMA Library, 2, 17, 19.

[43] Sir William Beveridge, *Social Insurance and Allied Services* (London: HMSO, 1942, Cmd. 6404), 8, 14, 120, 159.

premiums were better than services supported entirely by taxes because, having paid, people would demand their entitlement. If people paid additional premiums, they could obtain more medical care than the minimum to which mandatory insurance payments entitled them.[44]

Beveridge was uncomfortable about discussing health policy. Almost two decades earlier he had declined to serve on the Royal Commission on National Health Insurance, claiming that he had no direct knowledge of the subject. In 1942 he was eager to acknowledge an emerging consensus on the substance of postwar health policy but to leave to others a detailed proposal for a national health service.[45]

The experts to whom he deferred—the leaders of the medical profession and senior officials in the ministry—believed that what reputable doctors did was the proper standard of care. They were committed to an optimum rather than a minimum standard in health policy. A minimum requires that explicit limits be set—perhaps even that treatment sometimes be withheld. Like the doctors, Beveridge assumed that it would be unethical to withhold care deliberately from any person. But unlike the doctors, Beveridge repeatedly endorsed a policy of entitlement to a minimum set of services.

To avoid contradiction, Beveridge implied that the minimum would eventually become the optimum. The experts to whom he deferred could design a self-limiting health policy. If the standard of living in Britain improved, and citizens had access to increasingly effective services, their need for diagnosis and treatment would most likely decline. They would then demand fewer services and doctors would be compelled by their ethics to provide less treatment. Beveridge assumed, therefore, that while the cost of other forms of social insurance would increase by 50 percent over the next two decades, health costs would be stable because, he said, the number of cases requiring treatment would decline.[46]

[44] *Ibid.*, 11, 14, 120, 159, 160-161. *Cf.* T. H. Marshall, *Social Policy in the Twentieth Century* (London: Hutchinson University Library, 4th ed., 1975), 100, who distinguished between a "social security system . . . with its guarantee of a minimum and the NHS, with its promise of the optimum."

[45] José Harris, *William Beveridge* (Oxford: Clarendon Press, 1977), 352, 389. Harris noted (427) that "his assumption of a national health service directly reflected current thinking in the medical profession and Ministry of Health"; Beveridge, *Social Insurance*, 159-160, 162.

[46] *Ibid.*, 161, 105.

CONFLICT WITHIN CONSENSUS

Between 1943 and 1945, the ministry struggled to design policy for a postwar health service to implement the consensus described in Beveridge's report.[47] The debate among officials and interest groups about the distribution of power in a regionalized system was, however, increasingly acrimonious. Agreement on fundamentals made a national health service possible, but it did not resolve long-standing conflicts. Moreover, although the Conservative and Labour partners in the Government agreed that the policy emerging from extensive negotiations was a workable compromise, both parties, but especially Labour, had objections to it. As Lord Woolton, the minister for reconstruction, told Prime Minister Churchill, the compromise was much more favorable to the Conservative than to the Labour ministers.[48]

Agreement about the general outlines of postwar health policy was eroded by conflict about how hospitals should be governed and doctors paid. Members of each faction in the medical profession and among the laymen and women who governed hospitals as either officials of local authorities or members of voluntary boards had strong opinions on these issues.

The issues in conflict were discussed in 1943 by leaders of interest groups and senior civil servants at meetings held by the ministry to obtain advice about postwar policy. At the first meeting between the Representative Committee of the Medical Professions and officials of the ministry, the doctors described a postwar world in which central policies would be administered through regional bodies. They objected, however, to regional organizations that would place them under the control of local authorities.[49] During the same month, representatives of local authorities and voluntary hospitals,

[47] The consensus within the medical community was reinforced by public opinion. Two weeks after the Beveridge Report was published, the Gallup Poll reported that 95% of respondents had heard about it, with "overwhelming agreement" that the plan "should be put into effect." The proposal to make "doctors' and hospital services . . . free of charge to every person . . . was heartily endorsed" by respondents of every social class; 88% agreed, including 81% of the highest income group. However, only 53% of the public believed that the plan "would be put into effect." British Institute of Public Opinion, *The Beveridge Report and the Public* (London: the Institute, 1942), 3, 4, 8.

[48] CAB 124/244, PRO, Memorandum dated 10 February 1944. I am grateful to Rudolf Klein for this reference.

[49] "First Meeting with the Representative Committee of the Medical Profession," March 25, 1943, MH 77/26, PRO.

attending similar meetings, approved a tentative scheme for organizing services in regions of no fewer than 200,000 people.[50] The King Edward's Hospital Fund for London, a philanthropic foundation that represented the London teaching hospitals, declared that regions of appropriate size could remedy the haphazard distribution of hospitals. This was a euphemistic attack on regions confined to the boundaries of local authorities as well as on small voluntary hospitals.[51] Within the ministry, some officials proposed to create new regional boards, while others wanted to rely entirely on local authorities or to divide power between local government and voluntary hospital representatives on joint boards. The permanent secretary, Sir John Maude and the chief medical officer, Sir Wilson Jameson, still believed that a comprehensive health program should be a local government service.[52]

Following these meetings, a Government statement about the competing proposals for postwar health policy, issued as a White Paper in 1944, described considerable agreement among officials and interest groups and set the terms for subsequent negotiations. The White Paper recalled the history of recommendations about regionalization since the report of the Consultative Council chaired by Lord Dawson in 1920 and 1921. The Government, its authors said, now proposed to organize services in regions large enough to offer a full range of hospital and specialist services. Within these regions, hospitals should be managed by joint authorities—combining counties and county boroughs—which would contract for services with voluntary hospitals. The new health service would provide comprehensive medical care. Doctor and hospital services would be free to all, but no person or voluntary institution would be compelled to participate. Most GPs would continue to be paid by capitation. Local authorities would, however, maintain health centers staffed by salaried doctors.[53]

Agreement on a compromise plan seemed to be imminent, although general practitioners, consultants, medical officers of

[50] March 23, 1942, MH 77/26, PRO.
[51] The King's Fund proposal was published as *Coordination of Hospital Services* (London: The Fund, March 1943). The Nuffield Trust produced a more detailed plan, which was available to the ministry in draft in May as "Comprehensive Health Services." The Fund, the Trust, and the Hospitals Association discussed these plans with the ministry on May 14, 1943, MH 77/26; MH 80/34, PRO.
[52] "Second Meeting with the Representative Committee of the Medical Profession," April 15, 1943, MH 77/26, PRO.
[53] Ministry of Health and Department of Health for Scotland, *A National Health Service* (London: HMSO, 1944, Cmd. 6502), *passim*.

health, leaders of voluntary hospitals, and officials of local authorities still had much to complain about. An official committee on medical schools, for example, reporting a few months later, described considerable agreement about future policy. The committee reported that leaders of every faction in the medical profession endorsed its recommendation that the zones of influence of large teaching hospitals were the proper regional units for a postwar health service. Each of these units would, the committee recommended, consist of a parent teaching hospital, secondary hospitals, and clinics. General practitioners would participate in these units through a systematic process for referring patients.[54] The London County Council announced plans to establish its own medical school. There was general agreement, moreover, that voluntary teaching hospitals should retain their existing governing boards, in order to be independent of the regional authorities which would manage other services.

Early in 1945, after additional discussions between officials and leaders of interest groups, civil servants drafted legislation for submission to Parliament when the war ended. The Cabinet accepted the principles described in the White Paper and the subsequent compromises on details negotiated by the civil servants. The doctors believed that their concerns about money and autonomy had largely been resolved. Leaders of the BMA, the Royal Colleges, and the Society of Medical Officers of Health endorsed the draft legislation.[55] Spokesmen for the British Hospitals Association and King Edward's Hospital Fund for London believed that voluntary interests could adequately be protected on the joint boards that would plan services for hospital regions.[56] Most leaders of local authorities

[54] Ministry of Health, *Report of the Interdepartmental Committee on Medical Schools* (London: HMSO, 1944), 7, 8, 15-16.

[55] The agreement, however strained, was reflected in the press. An untitled, undated memorandum by "TFC," probably July 1944, noted that "no newspaper came out against" the White Paper, while most made positive statements. MH 80/27, PRO. A memorandum from A. N. Rucker to Lord Cherwell, chairman of the Cabinet Committee on Reconstruction, September 27, 1944, reported that all organizations agree that there should be "regional coordination of planning over, roughly, the areas of university influence," but noted that the voluntary hospitals quietly "disagreed strongly" with the power accorded to local authorities. MH 80/27, PRO. A meeting at the ministry with a "small group from the Medical Profession," on August 4, 1944, was summarized by Lord Dawson as agreeing that the government proposals were the "right practical solution at the present time." MH 77/30B, PRO.

[56] Counterproposals that accepted the basic framework of the White Paper were made by both organizations: "Hospitals in the National Health Service: Counterproposals of the British Hospitals Association," British Medical Journal Supplement,

were satisfied with their role in regional planning and administration and in governing municipal hospitals.[57]

Eight years earlier, the authors of the PEP *Report* had struggled with the tensions in the consensus about priorities; their successors were enthusiastic about the White Paper and the compromises that followed it. The new health service, they said, would promote further evolutionary change. The time had come, according to PEP, for general practice to change not only from individual effort to teamwork but also from private to public enterprise.[58]

Despite the agreement about the draft legislation, disputes persisted within the medical profession and among interest groups. The goals of consultants and general practitioners were in conflict. Lord Moran, speaking for the Royal College of Physicians, told the minister, Henry Willink, in January 1945, that the College felt more strongly about regions than about anything else in the White Paper.[59] Moran regarded regionalization as the means to preserve the independence of teaching hospitals, to enhance the negotiating power of consultants, and to diminish the power of local authorities. He said that every doctor should be part of a great university service.[60] BMA leaders were torn by their dislike for Moran's hierarchical imperialism on the one hand and their suspicion of local authorities on the other. The price of GPs' freedom from local govern-

---

August 26, 1944, ii: 45-46. "Voluntary Hospitals and the White Paper: Views of the King's Fund," *ibid.*, September 16, 1944, ii: 59-60.

The hospital associations had good reason to be confident of their influence. In the summer of 1944, the ministry agreed to make drafts of the Hospital Surveys "available in full to the bodies affected." MH 80/33, PRO. The interest groups received what the ministry described as "unexpurgated" copies of the survey reports. The only one of these copies I found was in the British Hospital Association Papers (in British Hospitals Contributory Schemes Association Papers, LSE); the survey for Sheffield. The draft implicitly recommended a nationalized hospital system. This recommendation was eliminated from the published survey (see page 8).

[57] Society of Medical Officers of Health, *The White Paper on a National Health Service* (London: SMOH, September 29, 1944).

[58] PEP, *Medical Care for Citizens* (London: Europa Publishers Ltd., September, 1944), 15.

[59] Lord Moran to Henry Willink, January 29, 1945, MH 77/119, PRO.

[60] Moran's comment about a "university service" was made more than a year later, in Consultant Services Committee, *A Consultant Service for the Nation* (London: Harrison and Sons, 1946), 21. He reported, however, that Churchill showed him the draft Conservative election manifesto in the Spring of 1945 (Lord Moran, *Winston Churchill. The Struggle for Survival, 1940-1965* (London: Constable, 1966, 251-252). A draft of that manifesto read, "The whole service must be so designed that in each area the growth is helped and guided by the influence of a university." The draft was attached to Cabinet Minutes on the NHS, June 6, 1945, MH 77/30A PRO.

ment, they feared, could be their subordination to consultants.[61]

Conflict outside the profession was less intense by the spring of 1945 because leaders of most groups assumed that a compromise had been achieved.[62] Local authority spokesmen now worried mainly about the details of relationships in the future between voluntary and municipal hospitals and among members of their medical staffs. Moreover, they believed that their interests were protected by senior officials of the ministry. Voluntary hospital leaders, confident that they had retained independence and would receive a perpetual subsidy, paid attention mainly to organizing and administering a comprehensive service.[63]

The voluntary interest groups were not united. The Nuffield Trust wanted to confer separately with the ministry because of what it considered its special relationship to both voluntary hospitals and local authorities.[64] The King's Fund was more committed to maintaining the independence of teaching hospitals than was the British Hospitals Association.[65] Staff members of voluntary hospitals and contributory health insurance schemes, their jobs in jeopardy if services were reorganized, were more anxious about the future than were members of governing boards. During the negotiations after publication of the White Paper, some employees of voluntary hospitals publicized complaints about the ministry's proposals that were sufficiently threatening for a senior civil servant to suggest starting a whispering campaign among press correspondents in order to counter them.[66]

Local authority leaders were also in some disarray. A few of them believed that a national health service should be created after changes were made in the boundaries of local authorities.[67] Spokesmen for counties, municipal boroughs, and the LCC disagreed, however, about what criteria new boundaries should meet. Many

[61] On GPs see Honigsbaum *The Division*, and Eckstein, *The English Health Service*, *passim*.

[62] "First Meeting with Representatives of County Councils Association and LCC," June 14, 1944, "Meeting with Association of Municipal Corporations," June 20, 1944, make plain the ministry's support for local authority control while raising questions about the capacity of smaller authorities to manage a service. MH 77/30B, PRO.

[63] Address of the President . . . Annual General Meeting, 21st September 1944. British Hospital Contributory Scheme Association Papers, LSE.

[64] W. M. Goodenough to E. J. Maude, April 25, 1944, MH 80/34, PRO.

[65] The Fund's advocacy for teaching hospitals is evident in its "Memorandum on the National Health Service," July 1944, MH 80/34, PRO.

[66] A. N. Rucker to J. Hawton, May 25, 1944, MH 80/34, PRO.

[67] Association of Municipal Corporations to Ministry, 18 May 1944; County Councils Associations to Ministry, 30 March 1944, MH 80/33, PRO.

county and borough leaders, for instance, disliked the assertion by leaders of the London County Council that large authorities were easier to administer.[68] But the local authorities had temporarily coalesced in order to reply to attacks by general practitioners and leaders of voluntary hospitals on their health services. As a member of the LCC had remarked a year earlier, the only real alternative to creating the health authorities proposed in the White Paper was a centralized national service.[69]

Several groups were dissatisfied with any compromise that preserved voluntary hospitals and forced local authorities to form joint boards with them. Within the ministry, senior officials—notably John Hawton, John Pater, and Sir Wilson Jameson—were gradually persuaded by the experience of the Emergency Medical Service that all hospitals should be nationalized and then administered in what they called natural regions.[70] The Trades Union Congress also preferred to incorporate voluntary institutions in a unified hospital system based on hospital regions that did not have political boundaries.[71]

By the end of the war, these disputes about health policy were about means rather than ends. Hierarchy, equity, and efficiency had become shared goals. Leaders of each interest group agreed that a national health service should array services in hierarchies and make them available to all citizens without direct charge, be financed mainly by the central government, offer free choice of doctors, and be committed to both preventing and curing illness. The groups disagreed about how to govern hospitals, how to coordinate hospitals with each other and with the ambulatory and home-care services of local government, and about how doctors should be paid and regulated.

In 1944, leaders of each group within the medical and hospital communities had expressed their preference for the means to achieve the goals they shared. In the summer of 1945, they were prepared to advocate their plans again if a new Government re-

[68] LCC draft reply to White Paper, April 1944, p. 32. The quotation was eliminated from the published version of the LCC position, in January 1945, to spare the political sensibilities of the smaller local authorities. MH 80/33, PRO.

[69] "Fourth Meeting Between Representatives of Local Authorities and the Officers of the Ministry." MH 77/26, PRO.

[70] The history of commitment to nationalization in the ministry and of John Hawton's role in it is Pater's most original contribution in *Making of the National Health Service*, 178-179.

[71] *Trades Union Congress*, Blackpool, 1944; *Government White Paper on a National Health Service, General Council Report.* Supplement, 11 (MH 80/27, PRO).

opened discussions about policy.[72] Leaders of the British Medical Association preferred regional hospital councils to represent public and voluntary interests and doctors. Spokesmen for the Society of Medical Officers of Health and the Socialist Medical Association wanted a single hospital system, based on reorganized local authorities. The leaders of the Medical Practitioners Union, speaking for just over 3,000 doctors, believed that all hospitals must be taken over by the ministry, and they regarded as nonsense the idea that services must be based on hospitals.[73] But the MPU also demanded a protected status for teaching hospitals. Some doctors still believed that a national health corporation was desirable.[74] Officials of the British Hospital Association, the King's Fund, and the Nuffield Trust proposed that voluntary interests be guaranteed representation on local health authorities.[75]

During the election campaign of 1945, each party took a position on organizing a future health service that was designed to attract the support of members of particular medical and hospital interest groups. The Conservative party accepted the agreements worked out by the ministry since the White Paper but made additional concessions to doctors after Labour left the coalition to contest the election. Liberals wanted local authorities to control voluntary hospitals in loosely organized regions. The Communist party advocated hospital committees, with members from all grades of health workers, to administer regions and individual institutions. Labour wanted to move gradually to public control through a unified system of admissions to hospitals.[76]

After the election, which was an overwhelming victory for Labour, how doctors would be paid was a much more controversial issue than how regions would be organized. Alone among the parties, Labour had consistently advocated that general practitioners be paid by salary rather than capitation or fees. Labour's public po-

[72] A notable summary of these views was James M. Mackintosh, *The Nation's Health, Target for Tomorrow*, vol. 5 (London: The Pilot Press, 1944), 48. Mackintosh also noted (47), "There is a broad similarity between the evolution of the health services in Britain and the United States."

[73] Medical Practitioners Union, "The Transition to a State Medical Service," August, 1942, MH 77/26, PRO. *Cf.* Honigsbaum, *The Division*, 280.

[74] Lord Dawson, for example, and various members of the BMA. See note 36, above. The concept had first been described in print by Dr. Stephen Taylor, a member of the Labour party, in "A Plan for British Hospitals," *The Lancet*, October 28, 1939, ii: 945-951.

[75] See above, note 56.

[76] Mackintosh, *Nation's Health, passim*.

sition on health policy during the war was articulated mainly by the Socialist Medical Association, which had long been committed to a full-time salaried medical service. But the leaders of the SMA, as they had indicated in the past, regarded salaried general practice as a lower priority than both guaranteeing universal entitlement to care and establishing regional hierarchies. Moreover, the leaders of the party, absorbed for six years in the affairs of the Coalition Government, had not yet taken a public position on how to administer a new health service.

In the summer of 1945 the Labour Government had only a few choices to make about the proposed national health service. The party's health policy had emerged over a generation. Its leaders, Clement Attlee, Ernest Bevin, and Herbert Morrison, had participated in confidential discussions about postwar health policy as members of the War Cabinet. The new minister of health, Aneurin Bevan, was briefed by civil servants who had been managing an Emergency Medical Service for six years and who had been planning a postwar health service for five.

The new Government was obligated, however, to reexamine the agreement about postwar policy that had been negotiated with leaders of medical, hospital, and local government interest groups. The Government took only a few political risks in pausing briefly to assess the compromise negotiated since 1944. The leaders of medical and voluntary hospital associations would object to changing what they had agreed to, but most of them were not Labour supporters. Leaders of the large municipal authorities had no political home outside the Labour party, and no reason to expect the party to damage their interests. Moreover, reassessment was appreciated by several groups within the Labour party. The members of the Socialist Medical Association wanted to advocate a salaried medical service. Officials of the Trades Union Congress bristled at the condescension of voluntary hospital governors and were indifferent to the administrative concerns of local government officials. In addition, most members of the general public were not interested in the issues of governance and autonomy that bothered doctors and hospital leaders. Forty-two percent of the respondents in a widely publicized poll were prepared to see voluntary hospitals taken over by either local authorities or the Ministry of Health.[77]

The Government's reconsideration of health policy was rapid and

---

[77] British Institute of Public Opinion, *The Nation's Health* (London: The Institute, Summer, 1944), 26.

was limited to problems of implementing a national health service. The Government embraced the goals of hierarchy, equity, and efficiency. In less than forty years, the priority of health policy had changed from preventing poverty to alleviating physical distress and then to providing all citizens with the means for care and cure. Prevention, once conceived mainly as measures to improve the general welfare—environment, nutrition, housing, and income—had been redefined to include discrete services provided by health professionals to individuals. Hierarchy in the organization of services was assumed to be an inevitable result of scientific and technical advance. Hierarchical relationships should be administered through regional networks of doctors, hospitals, and supporting services. When financial and geographic barriers to access by patients were removed or reduced, priorities for allocating resources within a national health service would, almost everyone agreed, be determined by the efficient application of the findings of medical science to the needs of individuals.

By 1945 these opinions were regarded as self-evident. They were shared by officials of central and local government, by doctors, and by hospital leaders. Politicians and newspaper proprietors accepted them. The general public, according to several polls, was overwhelmingly in favor of a comprehensive national health service available to all citizens. The experience of total war had, moreover, increased citizens' impatience to achieve a better standard of living—a more equitable distribution of the nation's resources. Sir William Beveridge, to the surprise of some political leaders, had articulated popular aspirations for equity in entitlement to medical care and social security as well as a consensus among experts.

In Britain, by the end of the war, powerful beliefs about how to organize medical services and how to distribute them to the public reinforced each other. Hierarchy, implemented through regionalization, was now generally agreed to be the precondition to achieving equity of access to services of appropriate quality. Ideas that were grounded in an interpretation of how medical science advanced and was most efficiently applied now reinforced ideas about the rights of citizens which were derived from political philosophy and from the experience of class conflict in peacetime and national solidarity in war.

VII

The Second World War
and Health Policy:
The United States, 1941-1946

THE ORGANIZATION of medicine for war influenced postwar health policy in the United States as it did in Britain. In 1932, Roger I. Lee, writing for the Committee on the Costs of Medical Care, had defined good medical care as what respected specialists did.[1] In 1945, as president of the AMA, Lee announced that his standard had changed from how leaders of the profession practiced to the extraordinary care given to fighting men.[2] The same year, President Harry S. Truman, announcing his support for health policy opposed by the AMA, declared that the armed forces provided the best medical and hospital care. Veterans and their dependents, he said, deserved adequate and comprehensive care.[3] This agreement about the implications of war for health policy facilitated the work of a coalition advocating policy to increase the supply of medical services, beginning with Federal subsidies to construct hospitals.

MILITARY MEDICINE AND CIVILIAN POLITICS, 1941-1945

According to the press, the United States won the war against wounds and disease long before it vanquished the Axis. Articles in newspapers and popular magazines proclaimed, for example, "New Medical Miracles Save Thousands in Battles," "All Out War on Germs," and "War Brings Healing Miracles."[4] As a result of the

[1] Roger I. Lee and Lewis Webster Jones, *The Fundamentals of Good Medical Care* (Chicago; University of Chicago Press, 1933), 6.

[2] Roger I. Lee, "What is Adequate Medical Care," *Journal of the American Medical Association*, December 8, 1945, 129: 990; *cf.* Edgar E. Robinson and Paul C. Edwards, eds., *The Memoirs of Ray Lyman Wilbur*, 621.

[3] Harry S. Truman, "Special Message to the Congress Recommending A Comprehensive Health Program" Public Papers of the Presidents of the U.S. April 12-December 31, 1945 (Washington, D.C.: USGPO, 1961), 490. *Cf.* Davis R. B. Ross, *Preparing for Ulysses: Politics and Veterans During World War II* (New York: Columbia University Press, 1969).

[4] Ross I. McIntire, "New Medical Miracles Save Thousands in Battle," November

war, a prominent doctor wrote, such innovations as antibiotics, blood plasma, and DDT would dominate peacetime medicine.[5] Photographs of medicine at war reinforced this point of view. *Life's* coverage of military medicine was a running story of hope. Its "Odyssey of a Wounded Soldier," for instance, arrayed images of a young man's progress from being wounded in Normandy through battlefield surgery, treatment with penicillin to fight infection, a comfortable convalescence, and a transatlantic flight home.[6]

As a result of their military experience, more doctors wanted to become specialists and to practice in groups. By 1943 almost half the physicians under the age of sixty-five who had been in private practice were in the armed forces. Most of these doctors had attended medical school after 1920 and thus had been instructed in basic sciences by full-time teachers and had received clinical training in accredited teaching hospitals. Most of them had been interns for a year and many also had some specialty training. Most lived in cities or large towns, though doctors from small towns and rural areas, who were eager to relocate, enlisted at the fastest rate. The armed forces gave certified specialists higher ranks and broader responsibilities than even the most experienced general practitioners. At the end of the war, thousands of doctors entered specialty training subsidized by the G.I. Bill of Rights. In a poll taken in 1945, 58 percent of military doctors who planned to enter private practice said that they preferred to practice in a group.[7]

1943, 136: 26-27, 108-109, 112; Sydney B. Self, "All Out War on Germs," *Science Digest* [condensed from the *Wall Street Journal*], December 1946, 10: 60-63; Justina Hill, "War Brings Healing Miracles," "*Science Digest*, March 1943, 13: 39-42. *Cf.*, "Atomic Healer: Men in White Aim Cyclotrons at Disease Instead of Armies," *Newsweek*, December 24, 1945, 26: 75.

[5] Iago Galston, "The New Life Savers," *Survey Graphic*, June 1945, 34: 292: Galston made similar claims in *Popular Science* in "Magic Drugs, Ingenious Instruments, Wider Knowledge Mark the Rapid Advancement of the Last Three Decades," December, 1943, 143: 82-84. E. L. Koos, surveying the population of a small town in upstate New York just after the war in the study that became *The Health of Regionville* (New York: Hafner, 1954, 1967), found that "The concept of the family doctor as one who provides medicine in the home and is a walking drugstore has had to be revised sharply. . . . The experiences of the war years and the expansion of the pharmacopoeia have both hastened this revision" (62).

[6] "Odyssey of George Cott, Casualty," *Life*, January 28, 1945, 18: 15-27; *cf.* "Capture of Naples," *Life*, October 18, 1943, 15: 34-35, where photojournalism combined medical and religious imagery.

[7] Harold C. Lueth, "Economic Aspects of Future Medical Practice," *Journal of the American Medical Association*, June 16, 1945, 128: 528-529, reported the poll. A useful contemporary survey of medical practice is Bernhard J. Stern, *American Medical Prac-*

New relationships between the federal government and health institutions were established as a result of the war. The government subsidized medical schools to accelerate the training of physicians and civilian hospitals to treat wounded servicemen. An Emergency Maternity and Infant Care program, administered by the United States Children's Bureau through the states, reimbursed voluntary hospitals for the costs of providing care to dependents of enlisted men.[8] Scientists in university and hospital laboratories developed drugs and equipment under federal contracts. In 1945, many of these contracts were converted into grants by the National Institutes of Health, which Congress had authorized a year earlier to fund research in universities, hospitals, and nonprofit research institutes.[9]

A new coalition of interest groups worked to maintain and extend these innovations in health policy after the war. This coalition, like the Committee of 430 in the previous decade, was led by academic doctors who were now joined by leaders of the American Hospital Association. Philanthropic foundations and the United States Public Health Service financed many of the coalition's activities. The leaders of the new coalition practiced the politics of consensus. They emphasized principles that had enthusiastic public support, and sought sponsors for their proposals among conservative politicians because liberals had no alternative to supporting increased public subsidy for medical care. They took advantage of the president's preoccupation with the war to obtain active support from the Public Health Service in the absence of explicit Administration policy. By 1945, the coalition's work had neutralized the most militant opponents of what was called socialized medicine by leaders of the AMA. Advocates of national health insurance could only complain that the coalition's program did not go far enough.

The coalition described its program in two reports prepared during the war. The New York Academy of Medicine organized a Committee on Medicine and the Changing Order, which was composed of prominent doctors and members of other health professions. The

tice in the Perspective of a Century (New York: The Commonwealth Fund, 1945). For half of American doctors in the armed forces see, "Doctor Shortage and Civilian Health in Wartime," Journal of the American Medical Association, September 25, 1943, 123: 214.

[8] Martha M. Eliot, "Experience with Administration of a Medical Care Program for Wives and Infants of Enlisted Men," American Journal of Public Health, January 1944, 34: 34-39.

[9] Stephen P. Strickland, Politics, Science and Dread Disease (Cambridge: Harvard University Press, 1972), 18-19.

committee issued a series of papers and books beginning in 1942.[10] The American Hospital Association created a Commission on Hospital Care, consisting of hospital trustees and managers and leading doctors, which issued studies and summaries of its work between 1943 and 1946.[11]

These reports were platforms rather than manifestos. Their purpose was to unite diverse, often conflicting constituencies. The authors of the reports endorsed group practice but only as one among several ways to achieve a desirable relationship between generalists and specialists. Both reports endorsed voluntary health insurance, but both also emphasized their authors' willingness to negotiate about preserving doctors' autonomy and consumers' choices under mandatory insurance. The authors carefully equivocated about whether there was or would soon be a shortage of doctors. The committee described the virtues of general practice but assumed that hospitals and specialists would offer diagnostic services and consultation to doctors who did not, and—it implied—should not, have hospital privileges. The commission complained about low wages in hospitals but avoided endorsing unions. Similarly, it deplored racism but accepted segregated hospitals.[12]

Both the committee and the commission, however, endorsed hierarchical regionalism as the fundamental principle of postwar policy. Proper regional organization would be achieved by subsidy and consensus rather than by coercion, their members agreed. Community and teaching hospitals should be linked in regional networks in order to distribute services more rationally and enhance their quality. Each of these networks should, however, be created voluntarily. Each would link health centers and other satellite institutions with a large teaching hospital. Although the principle of hierarchial regionalism was derived from the history of medical science, it must be adapted to the needs of each community. Hierarchical regionalism could best be promoted by a variety of measures, which included public subsidies to construct hospitals, private incentives to increase doctors' willingness to practice in underserved

[10] New York Academy of Medicine, Committee on Medicine and the Changing Order, *Medicine in the Changing Order* (New York: The Commonwealth Fund, 1947).

[11] Commission on Hospital Care, *Hospital Care in the United States* (New York: The Commonwealth Fund, 1947).

[12] *Medicine in the Changing Order, passim.*; the recommendations of the commission were published independently in A. C. Bachmeyer, "Problems Confronting American Hospitals," *Hospital Review*, 1945, Part II, 13-18.

areas, and federal grants to improve the states' services to the poor.[13]

During the war, philanthropic foundations and the United States Public Health Service helped to establish local coalitions of individuals committed to organizing medical care in regional hierarchies based on hospitals. The Kellogg Foundation and the Commonwealth Fund funded regional consortia of hospitals and programs to link medical school faculty and community doctors in Maine, Massachusetts, Michigan, New York, Tennessee, and Virginia.[14] Surgeon General Parran said that he looked forward to a system of university hospital centers feeding knowledge to other hospitals.[15] Two senior officials of the PHS, Vane Hoge and Joseph Mountin, proposed a theory of regionalization for hospital planning and construction and for training and distributing doctors.[16]

Most important, foundations and the PHS collaborated to mobilize support for federal legislation to build hospitals after the war. The Commission on Hospital Care was financed by the Commonwealth Fund, the Kellogg Foundation, and the National Foundation for Infantile Paralysis. In 1943, the commission and the PHS announced a joint program of assistance to states. Assuming that postwar legislation to construct hospitals would require surveys of existing facilities, the commission signed a contract with the PHS to anticipate federal survey requirements. Under this contract, the PHS assigned federal officials to state health departments to begin surveys under the auspices of the commission.[17]

---

[13] Ibid.; Medicine in the Changing Order, 90ff., 97, 222.

[14] A contemporary review of foundation activities in rural areas is in Frederick D. Mott and Milton I. Roemer, Rural Health and Medical Care (New York: McGraw Hill, 1948) 455-466; cf. Henry J. Southmayd and Geddes Smith, Small Community Hospitals (New York: The Commonwealth Fund, 1944).

[15] Furman, A Profile of the United States Public Health Service (Washington, D.C.: USGPO, 1955), 439

[16] Ibid., 415; Ralph C. Williams, The United States Public Health Service, 1798-1950 (Washington, D.C.: Commissioned Officers Association of the USPHS, 1951), 342, 346. Cf Milton I. Roemer and Robert C. Morris, "Hospital Regionalization in Perspective," Public Health Reports, October, 1959, 74: 918: "During World War II . . . the regionalization idea matured. . . ."

[17] George Bugbee provided a history in "An Address by George Bugbee," at the First Meeting of the Federal Hospital Council September 17-18, 1946, Washington, D.C. (Chicago: American Hospital Association, 1947). Hoge gave his version in V. N. Hoge, "The Hospital Survey and Construction Act," Public Health Reports, January 10, 1947, 62: 49-54. A recent paper purporting to be a history of these events has many errors of fact: Dan Feshbach, "What's Inside the Black Box . . . ," International

By the end of 1943, the American Hospital Association led a growing coalition advocating federal legislation to construct hospitals after the war. First the AHA had achieved agreement about the substance of legislation with the Catholic and Protestant Hospital Associations. Then the three hospital associations had obtained commitments to support this legislation from the American Medical Association, the American Federation of Labor, the Congress of Industrial Organizations, the Railroad Brotherhoods, the Farm Bureau Federation, the Farmers' Union, the Grange, and the General Federation of Women's Clubs.

In 1944, George Bugbee of the AHA and Vane Hoge of the PHS drafted and promoted a bill to construct hospitals. Bugbee circulated the draft bill to leaders of every faction in health politics. He suggested to Michael Davis, for example, that the coalition might be amenable to pressure from the militant reformers to expand its program.[18] Dr. Hoge had supervised surveys in twenty-two states by the end of 1945 and helped eighteen states draft laws that would enable them to administer a program to plan and construct hospitals. In 1943 he had told an audience of hospital staff and trustees at a national meeting that the PHS estimated an immediate postwar need of $2 billion to build new hospitals and replace older ones. He called military medicine the most important influence creating future demand for hospital care. To meet this demand, he said, hospital leaders should link the campaign for construction subsidies with aggressive efforts to obtain reimbursement from third-party payers for the full cost of each patient's care.[19]

In July 1944, Surgeon General Parran, explained the goals of the coalition to Senator Claude Pepper's subcommittee on Wartime

---

Journal of Health Services, no. 2, 1979, 9: 313-339. *Cf.* Paul Starr, *The Social Transformation of American Medicine* (New York: Basic Books, 1982), 347-351. For the mobilization of a constituency in behalf of federal funding for mental health services and research during the same months, see Jeanne L. Brand, "The National Mental Health Act of 1946: A Retrospect," *Bulletin of the History of Medicine*, May-June 1965, 39: 231-245.

[18] George Bugbee to Michael W. Davis, December 30, 1944. Davis Papers, M-1, New York Academy of Medicine. George Bugbee, Letter to "Members of Hospital Administrators Correspondence Club," November 10, 1948, Mimeographed, Davis Papers, M-1.

[19] V. M. Hoge, "Add Another Two Billions for 'Adequate' Future Plant," *Hospitals*, December 1943, 17: 21-24. *Cf.* Mott and Roemer, *Rural Health*, 498, for State planning activities prior to passage of the Hill-Burton Act. The alliance between the USPHS and the AHA is documented in memoranda between Hoge and Parran in USPHS, General Classified Records, Surgeon General's Files, Box 92, National Archives of the United States.

Health and Education. After the war, Parran said, people would demand more physicians and hospital care, which they would purchase through some form of prepayment. The immediate task, however, was to build adequate facilities, taking advantage of the existing investment in voluntary hospitals. Federal grants to build hospitals, unlike grants from the New Deal public works programs, should be made to states rather than to local governments or hospitals themselves. Surveys and plans, coordinated by a single agency in each state, should precede federal grants. Doctors need not fear such a program, which would complement their specialized knowledge.[20] Parran's testimony, in which he recanted his assertion of federal authority and local inadequacy in 1940, was widely circulated by the American Hospital Association.[21]

The Public Health Service provided analytical as well as political support for the coalition's agenda. Writing in a PHS bulletin in 1944, Hoge, Mountin, and statistician Elliott Pennell divided the nation into 126 regions of 300,000 people for whom health care should be organized by local initiative into hierarchies dominated by hospitals. The base hospital in each of these regions would be linked to 538 district hospitals—almost half of which were yet to be built—and 106 health centers to serve isolated areas. Base hospitals should be associated, wherever practicable, with medical schools. The nation needed 165,000 new hospital beds, a conclusion the authors based on the standard of adequacy that Roger I. Lee and Lewis Webster Jones had derived a decade earlier in their research for the CCMC using what were now said to be strictly medical factors.[22]

The Commission on Hospital Care also used a formula to determine the need for hospital beds. Substituting mortality for morbidity in the Lee-Jones equation, the commission determined that, under the best medical practice, an average of 250 days of hospitalization was required for each death. For the near future, when only

[20] Thomas Parran, Testimony to U.S. Senate, Subcommittee on Wartime Health and Education, July 12, 1944; reprinted in *Hospitals*, August 1944, 18: 41ff., and in A. C. Bachmeyer and Gerhard Hartmen, eds., *Hospital Trends and Developments 1940-46* (New York: The Commonwealth Fund, 1948).

[21] *Cf.* Thomas Parran's recantation, "More Health Care Is Inevitable," *Hospitals*, October 1943, 17: 48-51. Parran later insisted that "he did not originate this plan of great university hospital centers radiating out to smaller hospitals but got it from fellow officers of the PHS" (Furman, *A Profile*, 447).

[22] Federal Security Agency, United States Public Health Service, *Health Service Areas: Requirements for General Hospitals and Health Centers* (Public Health Bulletin no. 292) (Washington, D.C.: USGPO, 1945), 5-6.

half the population would die in hospitals, the proper ratio of beds to population should be 5:1000.[23]

The American Medical Association endorsed the goals of the new coalition. In 1945, its Committee on Postwar Service asserted that more doctors were needed to care for civilians, veterans, citizens of liberated countries, and peacetime military forces. Growing enrollment in health insurance plans, moreover, was increasing the demand for medical care.[24] A few months later, the House of Delegates overwhelmingly supported a proposal by Paul Hawley, chief medical officer of the Veterans' Administration, to link medical schools and Veterans' Hospitals on a regional basis.[25]

The leaders of the coalition promoting legislation to build new hospitals were sensitive to the distribution of power in national politics at the end of the war. Congress was dominated by conservative Democrats and Republicans who shaped domestic policy to satisfy the interests and aspirations of the people who elected them; middle-class whites who lived in rural areas, small towns, and middle-sized cities in the Middle West and the South. These conservative congressional leaders had no incentive to support the proposals to subsidize medical care, housing, transportation, or employment that were advocated by the minority of their colleagues elected from districts or states with large working-class and labor union constituencies.[26]

Both Roosevelt and Truman contributed more rhetoric than presidential power on behalf of health policy. During the 1944 election campaign, presidential assistant Harry Hopkins, briefly resuming his prewar role as emissary to social reformers, told Michael Davis that the president was ready to advocate national health insur-

[23] *Hospital Care in the U.S.*, 298-301.

[24] "Medicine and the War: The Supply of Medical Students and Physicians," memorandum presented on June 4, 1945 to President Harry S. Truman by a special committee of the Committee on Postwar Medical Service [AMA], *Journal of the American Medical Association*, July 21, 1945, 128: 884. *Cf.* Maxine Davis, "Doctor Shortage," *Saturday Evening Post*, December 12, 1942, 215: 22, 96-98; *cf.* "Rural Health: Vanishing Country M.D.s," *Newsweek*, March 24, 1947, 29: 58, 59-60.

[25] Vernon W. Lippard, *A Half Century of American Medical Education* (New York: Josiah Macy, Jr., Foundation, 1974), 67: "the three influences that had the most telling effect on medical education in the twentieth century were the Flexner Report, the entry of the Federal government into the support of medical research and the establishment of a close relationship between veterans' hospitals and their neighboring medical schools."

[26] For the Conservative Coalition see Richard Polenberg, *War and Society: The United States 1941-1945* (Westport: Greenwood Press, 1972), Chapters III-IV.

ance.[27] But other reformers within the Administration, Arthur Altmeyer of the Social Security Board, for example, doubted Roosevelt's commitment to insurance.[28] Harry Truman spoke forcefully in
favor of a comprehensive health program based on health insurance. But Truman's words were intended mainly to solicit support
from liberals without losing the allegiance of moderates. According
to one historian, he was reluctant to endorse the bills introduced in
Congress to implement his health program.[29]

The coalition also took advantage of the temporary absence of coordination of domestic social policy in the executive branch. The authority of the Bureau of the Budget was diminished during the war,
when it lost many of its responsibilities to the Office of War Mobilization. As a result, until 1947, officials of domestic agencies were
freer than they had been in the 1930s to advocate policies without
obtaining central clearance for them.[30] The Public Health Service,
for example, collaborated with interest groups and congressional
committees to shape a bill to construct hospitals that was independent of the comprehensive health program announced by the President.

PHS staff members, moreover, retained close relationships with
officials of state government, where many of them had once
worked. Many state officials were enraged by New Deal economic
and social legislation that authorized direct grants to county and
city government. Their colleagues in the PHS were determined that
national health policy would not bypass the states.[31]

THE HILL-BURTON ACT, 1945-1946

The coalition of groups promoting the Hospital Survey and Construction bill introduced in Congress in 1945 was unified only by its
belief that the proper way to disseminate the results of the progress
of medicine was through hospitals, which were the dominant med-

[27] Monte M. Poen, *Harry S. Truman Versus the Medical Lobby* (Columbia: University
of Missouri Press, 1979), 49-50.

[28] Arthur J. Altmeyer, *The Formative Years of Social Security* (Madison: University of
Wisconsin Press, 1966) *passim.*

[29] Poen, *Harry S. Truman, passim.*

[30] Richard E. Neustadt, "Presidency and Legislation: The Growth of Central Clearance," *The American Political Science Review,* September 1954, 48: 641-671.

[31] Bugbee, "An Address"; Daniel Hirshfield, *The Lost Reform* (Cambridge: Harvard
University Press, 1970), *passim.*: Poen, *Harry S. Truman, passim.*; Furman, *A Profile,
passim.*

ical institutions in particular geographic areas. Coalition leaders in Congress, the Public Health Service, and the American Hospital Association understood that, as a result of lingering bitterness and suspicion from past conflicts between organized medicine and the vanguard of reform, they could create, at best, a fragile coalition to support limited goals. In order to pass legislation, they had to seek allies among Americans who believed that social policy should be made by local economic and political elites rather than by the national groups proposing to expand the general welfare state.

Some members of the coalition wanted much more than the leaders did, however. Organized labor, officials of the United States Social Security Board, and a few liberal congressmen advocated a comprehensive program of health services that would be paid for by national health insurance. The members of the three national hospital associations—American, Catholic, and Protestant—wanted their institutions to be reimbursed for the care they provided to the indigent. Other members of the coalition, particularly leaders of the American Medical Association, the United States Chamber of Commerce, and the Farm Bureau Federation hoped that subsidies for hospital construction would be an isolated policy rather than the first step in a health program whether it would be limited or comprehensive.

The leaders of the coalition advocating hospital subsidy needed to mollify the labor leaders and liberal congressmen who advocated national health insurance. The liberals were, however, considerably less of a threat to the viability of the coalition than was organized medicine. Liberals would not oppose subsidies for hospital construction, which they had advocated for a decade. All they could do in 1945 was complain that a hospital construction program was only an installment on national health policy and ask for assurances that a broader program would be discussed. In 1938, members of the vanguard of reform drafted legislation and orchestrated hearings on measures to implement the National Health Program, which included subsidies for hospital construction. In the campaign for what became the Hill-Burton Act, they were merely another interest group. The substance and the timing of political action were controlled by men who were careful to limit their commitment, in public at least, to subsidies for hospitals.

The leaders of the coalition promoting the hospital construction bill had to persuade doctors that state and regional planning and coordination did not threaten their autonomy. Officials of the American Hospital Association and the Public Health Service agreed that regions, in which district hospitals were linked to base or teaching institutions, were the proper units for organizing services. But leaders of the AMA would passionately oppose any proposal that threatened to impose a hierarchy of doctors and hospitals. If the leaders of the AMA and the state medical societies believed that the hospital construction bill would change the way medical care was organized and financed, they would try to intimidate leaders of hospital associations, officials of state governments, and congressmen until they opposed it.

The supporters of the bill repeatedly assured doctors that the federal government would not use hospital subsidies to reorganize the practice of medicine. They argued that hospitals were effective because of what doctors were achieving. Constructing more hospitals would simply give more people access to the results of advancing medical science. Unlike the majority of the Committee on the Costs of Medical Care or the members of the Interdepartmental Committee on Health and Welfare, the promoters of subsidized hospital construction argued that the work of ordinary doctors exemplified medical progress. They included no elusive goal of positive health in their legislation. Moreover, they deemphasized the statements about hierarchy and regionalism that Public Health Service officials had made the year before when documenting the shortage of beds. The vanguard of reform in the 1930s used "lag" as their metaphor; the coalition promoting hospital construction changed it to "gaps," which could be closed by investing public and private funds to increase the supply of services.[32]

Leaders of the coalition were explicit about the importance of reassuring doctors. George Bugbee, who managed the campaign for the bill as a staff member of the American Hospital Association, believed that promoters of new health policy must be modest about what it could achieve. According to Bugbee, the vanguard of reform threatened doctors because its members raised false expectations among the public about the health, wealth, and happiness that doctors could provide. The only practical goal of policy, he urged, was greater access to hospitals. How relationships among doctors were organized and regulated and how care was paid for were, he implied, controversial issues that should be avoided.[33]

This strategy—affirming that hospitals were effective and reas-

[32] An example of the coalition's approach to mobilization was a trip by Bugbee to Knoxville, Tennessee, during four days in early April 1946, described in "Hospital Survey and Construction Bill," *Journal of the Tennessee Medical Association*, May 1946, 39: 166-168.

[33] George Bugbee, Letter to Members of Hospital Administrators Correspondence Club, November 10, 1948, Michael Davis Papers, M-1.

suring doctors that medical care was properly organized—was used to speed the hospital construction bill through Congress. The bill was introduced on a bipartisan basis. Its initial sponsors, Senators Lister Hill of Alabama and Harold H. Burton of Ohio, were members of the Senate's ruling coalition who appealed to different interest groups. Hill, who was the son of a doctor and had been named for the great nineteenth-century surgeon Joseph Lister, supported the economic program of the New Deal but was proponent of states' rights in education, civil rights, and the organization of medical services.[34] Burton, a moderate Republican, spent most of his political career in local government in Cleveland, where he had taken a non-doctrinaire approach to policy.[35] When Burton was appointed to the Supreme Court in 1945 by President Truman, as a result of their friendship when Truman was in the Senate, Robert A. Taft, his senior colleague from Ohio, became the Republican floor manager of the hospital construction bill. Taft had been interested in health policy since his college days as a student of Irving Fisher's at Yale and was active in hospital philanthropy in Cincinnati.[36]

Surgeon General Thomas Parran was the most visible federal official during congressional hearings on the Hill-Burton program. He repeatedly reassured congressmen and representatives of interest groups that, despite occasional White House rhetoric about national health insurance, this bill was not the first step toward it. Parran had learned from the failure of the National Health Program that public subsidy for medical care could increase only if those promoting it avoided open conflict. During the hearings, he frequently signaled the willingness of the executive branch to accommodate to the wishes of doctors and hospital leaders. Thus he formally regretted that he could not endorse the bill because there was no official policy yet on how it related to the President's program, and then accepted suggestions by the bill's supporters for changes in the way the PHS would administer it.[37] By calling attention to the White House's distraction by the war and to the temporary suspension of

[34] Stephen Strickland, *Politics, Science, and Dread Disease* (Cambridge: Harvard University Press, 1972), chapter I.

[35] Richard Kirkendall, "Harold Burton," in Leon Friedman and Fred C. Israel, eds., *The Justices of the United States Supreme Court* (New York: R. R. Bowker, 1969), 1617-2636.

[36] James T. Patterson, *Mr. Republican* (Boston: Houghton Mifflin Co., 1972), 14-15, 16, 41, 244.

[37] *Hospital Construction Act*, Hearings Before the Committee on Education and Labor, United States Senate, Seventy-ninth Congress, First Session, on S. 191, February 26, 27, 28, March 12, 14, 1945, 53, 76.

the Bureau of the Budget's role in legislative clearance, Parran implied that he agreed that policy for medical care should be a result of consensus among powerful interest groups. The PHS had become a participant in shaping that consensus: an agency, like most others in Washington, representing its clientele.

The organizers of the publicity that accompanied hearings and debate on the hospital construction bill chose tactics similar to those used by the AMA in its campaigns against comprehensive health legislation. Familiar tactics were reassuring. For instance, the leaders of the coalition promoting Hill-Burton behaved as if their success was in jeopardy. They distributed form letters for hospital trustees and doctors to personalize and send to their congressmen. Editorial writers in the medical and hospital press endorsed the bill fervently and frequently.

The organizers of the coalition used the Senate hearings to publicize the breadth of support for the bill and to suggest amendments that would reassure its more conservative supporters. The extent to which the hearings were contrived was made plain on the first day, when the president of the American Hospital Association formally introduced Bugbee to the people with whom he had worked closely for almost two years. Each organization in the coalition then gave the testimony expected of it. The Catholic Hospital Association even deemphasized the Church's fears about government intrusion into spiritual affairs.[38]

A few liberal senators, though supporting the bill, expressed reservations about it. Senator Claude Pepper of Florida, for example, insisted that hospital construction was merely preliminary to a comprehensive insurance plan. He claimed that the American Hospital Association, Surgeon General Parran, and even Morris Fishbein had recently agreed that the construction program was only the first step in a larger program.[39]

Senator Taft, in contrast, articulated conservatives' fear that the bill would promote both the haphazard growth of hospitals and federal power to coerce the states. He criticized the bill as, in his words, a wide open delegation to the surgeon general to use a spurious standard to construct as many beds as necessary. Taft said that he expected delegations from hospitals in Cincinnati and other cities to visit Washington demanding funds to double the size of their

[38] *Ibid., passim.* Organizational misgivings were buried in professional journals and were not displayed at the hearings. For example, Alphonse M. Schwitalla, S.J. "The Hospital Construction Act," *Hospital Progress*, December 1945, 26: 390-342.

[39] *Ibid.*, 64-65.

institutions. But Taft, as an advocate of the bill, was eager to reassure restless doctors. He denied the liberals' contention that the medical system was inadequate. The federal government's interest in medical care, he said, using the new metaphor, was merely to close the gaps.[40]

The leaders of the coalition promoting the bill were eager to mollify the members of the constituencies represented by both Pepper and Taft. Replying to Pepper's endorsement of comprehensive insurance, Parran minimized the need for public subsidy of hospital care. The number of people for whom hospital costs were paid by public agencies had, he claimed, declined since the Depression. Moreover, insurance against hospital and other medical costs would reduce the problem of care for the indigent. Parran had not, however, intended to imply that he still endorsed national health insurance. In reply to a subsequent question, he said that he expected that the requirement in the construction bill that hospitals have adequate operating funds would stimulate the expansion of Blue Cross plans. Parran also accepted Taft's amendments to the bill, agreeing to limit subsidies to large urban hospitals and to reduce the regulatory authority proposed for the PHS in the bill. States, he also agreed, must share the costs of construction and should not be permitted to receive subsidies to build or expand hospitals in areas that exceeded 4.5 beds per thousand population.[41]

The tone of Senate debate on the bill resembled that of the hearings. In his opening speech, Lister Hill declared that hospitals were the proper focus of health policy. Hospitals were complex technical machines, he said, which employed the latest scientific diagnostic aids, preventive and curative measures, and professional skills. They were, he continued, necessary for the practice of modern medicine. Although he could not attribute all the improvements in national health to more and better hospitals, they were, he insisted, a major factor.[42]

Taft and Hill emphasized the acceptability of the bill to every faction in the Senate except such doctrinaire liberals as Pepper, Robert

[40] *Ibid.*, 21, 26, 67, 77. Taft's views on social policy have been taken seriously by only a few scholars, notably Patterson. Frank J. Thompson, *Health Policy and the Bureaucracy: Politics and Implementation* (Cambridge: M.I.T. Press., 1981), argues that the requirement of ratios in the law "revealed [Taft's] sensitivity to the limits of development or growth" (31). Taft was more worried about arbitrariness than he was about oversupply.

[41] Senate Hearings, 66, 76, 89-90.

[42] *Congressional Record*, U.S. Senate, 79th Congress, First Session, vol. 91, December 10, 11, 1945: 11713-11714.

Wagner of New York, and Thomas Murray of Montana. Hill noted that the bill recognized the disparity in wealth among the states, gave special consideration to rural areas and communities with many low-income inhabitants, and encouraged states and localities to assume responsibility for the program. Local responsibility meant, he said, control by the people who provided services. Taft reminded his colleagues that the bill forced the states to take responsibility for the rights they cherished by requiring them to license and regulate hospitals in exchange for federal grants. As a Democrat, Hill was respectful of the president's comprehensive health program. Taft, after a partisan attack on the president's program, asserted that New Dealers, economic conservatives, and even opponents of an activist foreign policy should support the hospital bill. But Taft also kept the promises the organizers of the Hill-Burton coalition had made to liberals, proclaiming his willingness to support additional bills to subsidize health services.[43]

Liberal supporters of the bill used the debate as another opportunity to assert their views. Senator Wagner deplored policy that subsidized hospital construction but did not help people to pay the costs of hospital services. Senator Murray proposed amendments to strengthen federal power at the expense of the states and to prohibit discrimination against doctors because of either their race or desire to practice in groups. Both of Murray's amendments were defeated. Moreover, the director of the Bureau of the Budget had undercut the liberals' claim to speak on behalf of the president's health program by limiting his comments on the bill to minor technical objections to the role of the proposed Federal Hospital Council.[44]

The liberals were overpowered by a coalition that supported unprecedented federal expenditures for medical care but avoided the issues that had, for a generation, polarized debate about health policy. As Senator Johnston declared near the end of the debate, the desirability of a high standard of health was not controversial.[45]

The House acted promptly on the bill. Committee hearings were a reprise of those before the Senate committee.[46] Liberals, having stated their agenda in the Senate, refrained from proposing amendments that were sure to be defeated. Only four days after the House

[43] *Ibid.*, 11715-11716.

[44] *Ibid.*, 11717, 11719, 11795.

[45] *Ibid.*, 11701.

[46] *Hospital Construction Act*, Hearings Before a Subcommittee of the Committee on Interstate and Foreign Commerce, House of Representatives. 79th Congress, 2nd Session, S. 191. March 7, 8, 19, 11, 12, 13, 1946.

vote, a conference committee resolved the few differences in the two versions of the bill. John McCormack, the House majority leader, praised the coalition supporting the bill, observing that this was the first time he had ever seen such unanimity on health policy.[47] On July 30, 1946, the bill was sent to President Truman, who promptly signed it rather than holding it hostage for the passage of his comprehensive health program.[48]

The provisions of the Hill-Burton Act expressed a consensus about the proper role of government in American society as well as agreement about the centrality of hospitals in health policy. In 1946, the Americans who were most active in local and state affairs, who managed most business and industry, and who led civic and philanthropic organizations, believed that sovereignty ought to be decentralized. Hospitals, like schools, should be locally conceived and constructed, they asserted. They should be built and operated, it followed, with funds from either philanthropy, secular or religious, or local tax revenues, supplemented by federal grants that set few conditions. State governments should, they agreed, build and operate teaching hospitals for state university medical schools and institutions for poor people afflicted with chronic physical and mental illness.

According to the consensus, the federal government should provide resources to the states, which would distribute them to cities and counties. Some communities were too poor, and others were too thinly populated to organize hospitals without assistance, as Taft had emphasized in the Senate debate on the Hill-Burton Act. Some states lacked funds or expertise or incentive to build and regulate hospitals in the public interest, as Surgeon General Parran had testified. The federal government should assist all the states, but the poorer states more generously, to construct hospitals, as a majority of both houses of Congress had agreed. The federal government and the states should, in sum, set standards for hospital facilities and services but not interfere with local beliefs and politics.

The Hill-Burton Act decentralized control over hospital policy to settings in which state and local leaders exercised decisive influence. Doctors and business executives who complained about government interference were antifederal rather than antigovernment. They opposed rules they could not control. Doctors and their allies dominated the state boards and agencies that licensed professionals

[47] *Congressional Record*, House of Representatives, 79th Congress, 2nd Session, vol. 92, July 26, 1946: 10209.

[48] Poen, *Harry S. Truman*, 71.

and regulated hospitals and they enjoyed cordial relationships with state legislative leaders. Moreover, because the Hill-Burton Act mandated that construction subsidies be administered by a single agency in each state, leaders of hospital and medical groups were now empowered to reorganize state government to their satisfaction.

The Hill-Burton Act also decentralized the opportunity to organize regional hierarchies of hospitals. Leaders of the coalition promoting federal subsidy for hospital construction had avoided using arguments or legislative language that some doctors might perceive as threatening to reorganize medical care. The Committee on Medicine and the Changing Order and the Commission on Hospital Care had insisted that the hospitals in each region should be the organizational base for unique, locally devised hierarchies. Surgeon General Parran had even recanted his earlier abrasive statements about the necessity of hierarchy. But the desirability of hierarchical regionalism remained a fundamental assumption of many Public Health Service and state officials, hospital industry leaders, and academic doctors. Henceforth regional hierarchies would be created and strengthened as a result of the ability of local coalitions to achieve consensus and obtain subsidies from the Hill-Burton program as well as from state and philanthropic sources.

In 1946, the United States had, for the first time, a national health program for the general population. By the end of the Truman Administration, in 1952, despite the defeat of the president's comprehensive health policy, 88,000 new beds had been added to 1000 hospitals at a cost of $1.4 billion.[49] After three decades of stalemate, the politics of shared beliefs had created the preconditions for the politics of self-interest.

[49] Marion Ashley Buck, "An American Experiment, Cooperation for Health: A Study of the Hill-Burton Hospital Construction Act of 1946" (unpublished Ph.D. dissertation, Harvard University, 1953), 179; *cf.* Judith R. Lave and Lester B. Lave, *The Hospital Construction Act: An Evaluation of the Hill-Burton Program, 1948-1973* (Washington, D.C.: American Enterprise Institute, 1974).

VIII

Establishing the National Health Service:
Britain, 1946-1951

THE NATIONAL HEALTH SERVICE, established in 1946, reorganized but did not radically transform medical care in Britain. By the end of the war, the majority of employed workers were covered by National Health Insurance. Private insurance plans paid for doctors' services to most other people, including many dependents of workers covered by NHI. Many people had private hospital insurance. In the 1930s, many public hospitals, subsidized by local authorities, began to compete with the voluntaries. General practitioners earned most of their income from capitation payments. After 1939, consultants were salaried by the Emergency Hospital Service. Under the EHS, moreover, local authorities temporarily lost control of public hospitals but continued to provide clinic and home services for women, children, and the chronically ill.[1]

However, many people perceived the NHS as discontinuous with the past. Unlike Americans in the 1940s, who enacted national health policies in order to increase the supply of services justified by science, the British believed that the NHS was desirable because it was a centralized solution to broad social problems. The NHS quickly became a symbol of the more equitable social policy for which, many Britons believed, the war had been fought. Moreover, the NHS became a source of national pride in a country exhausted by war, its empire and thus its protected markets dissolving, its wealth depleted, its industrial plant and labor force increasingly obsolete. The achievements of the NHS were seen, moreover, as a contrast to postwar austerity—to food rationing that persisted until 1954 and shortages of fuel in the hard winters of the late 1940s.

THE POLITICS OF SHARED BELIEFS, 1946-1948

The bill to establish the National Health Service, which was presented to Parliament by the Government early in 1946, incorporated

[1] *The Lancet*, for example, commented in 1946 that the National Health Service "derives much more from the long discussions between the medical profession and the

most of the compromises reached during the previous two years. These compromises were made possible by a consensus that had emerged since the First World War. The major change imposed by the new Government was nationalizing voluntary and local authority hospitals. But only financing was to be centralized. The Government intended to delegate operating authority for its hospitals to regional health boards and management committees whose members would be the same people who had set policy when the institutions were voluntary or were administered by local authorities.

The decision to nationalize the voluntary hospitals was not a dramatic break with the past. For a generation, voluntary hospitals had relied on appropriations by the central government and subsidies from local authorities.[2] In 1918, a vice president of the British Hospitals Association had reassured his colleagues that voluntary effort was entirely consistent with public financing.[3] Since 1939 consultants had learned from the EHS that national management of hospitals enabled them to increase their control over administrative decisions.

Unlike the consultants, who were pleased by the proposed NHS, many general practitioners doubted the sincerity of the Government's commitment that they would continue to be independent contractors deriving their income from fees and capitation payments. GPs feared salaried status, not central government subsidy of medical care: 90 percent of them attended patients covered by National Health Insurance.[4] Before 1945, the Labour party, whose health policy was articulated by the Socialist Medical Association, advocated a salaried medical service. Moreover, the new minister of health, Aneurin Bevan, was abrasive and militantly class conscious. When the Coalition Government announced its commitment to a national hospital policy in 1941, Bevan had described voluntary hospitals to Parliament as repugnant to the conscience of the pub-

---

Ministry of Health than it does from any doctrinaire ideas of the present Minister's political party." Quoted in Gordon Forsyth, *Doctors and State Medicine* (London: Pitman Medical Publishing Company, 1966), 1.

[2] Forsyth, *Doctors and State Medicine*, 91, noted that between 1938 and 1947 fees from public authorities increased from 8% to 45% of voluntary hospitals' revenues while donations fell from 33% to 16%.

[3] *Report of the Annual Meeting and Conference in Reference to the Proposed Creation of a Ministry of Health*, March 18, 1918, 9. British Hospitals Association; British Hospitals Contributory Schemes Association Papers, British Library of Political and Social Science.

[4] John Powell Martin, *Social Aspects of Prescribing* (Melbourne: Heinemann, 1957), 5.

lic.[5] Early in 1946, moreover, he said that the time was not "ripe" for a salaried medical service, a remark which many general practitioners interpreted as a threat to change their status at a later date.[6]

Bevan was, however, strongly committed to increasing expenditures for health services, not to a particular policy for paying doctors. In the 1920s, as a member of the governing committee of a workmen's medical aid society in the Welsh coalfields, he demanded more doctor and hospital services.[7] In his first speech to a medical audience after becoming a minister, he asserted that the Ministry of Health should enable the medical profession to use the most modern technology.[8] Although he admired the achievements of preventive medicine, he preferred to promote the health of individuals rather than of populations. Health policy, he wrote a few years later, should address the suffering of individuals rather than seek the greatest good for the greatest number.[9] Bevan recommended nationalizing the hospitals in 1946, but probably not because of socialist doctrine. His goal was to provide curative services more equitably throughout the nation.[10]

Bevan may also have chosen to recommend nationalizing the hospitals as the result of advice about efficient administration he received from civil servants in the Ministry of Health. His taste for good food and drink and fondness for hyperbole encouraged later speculation that his views about consultants and hospitals were shaped by dinners at Prunier's restaurant with Lord Moran, president of the Royal College of Physicians.[11] In August 1945, however, John Hawton, the civil servant who had administered the Emergency Hospital Service and drafted the 1944 White Paper on postwar health policy, recommended that the Government nationalize the hospitals and manage them through appointed regional

[5] Hansard, *Parliamentary Debates*, 5th Series, vol. 374, House of Commons, October 9, 1941, col. 1119.

[6] Michael Foot, *Aneurin Bevan: A Biography*, vol. 2 (New York: Atheneum, 1974), 104ff.

[7] Foot, *Aneurin Bevan*, vol. 1 (New York: Atheneum, 1963), 45; "Where Bevan Got his National Health Plan," *Picture Post*, April 27, 1946, 30: 20-21 (the Tredegar Medical Aid Society).

[8] Foot, *Aneurin Bevan*, vol. II, 119.

[9] Aneurin Bevan, *In Place of Fear* (London: Heinemann, 1952), 73, 167-168.

[10] M. J. Buxton and R. E. Klein, *Allocating Health Resources: A Commentary on the Report of the Resource Allocation Working Party*, Research Paper no. 3, Royal Commission on the National Health Service (London: HMSO, 1978).

[11] Bevan himself, in later years, occasionally encouraged this impression, according to a personal communication from Brian Abel-Smith.

boards.[12] Wilson Jameson, the chief medical officer, apparently supported Hawton's recommendation, which was opposed by other senior officials.[13] By late September, Bevan had decided in favor of nationalization.[14]

Bevan's decision to nationalize public as well as voluntary hospitals surprised and distressed many Labour supporters. Many of the local authority hospitals had been established or modernized by County or Borough Councils dominated by Labour. Like many voluntary hospital governors, however, some Labour leaders with roots in local government were sympathetic to central control. For example, two years earlier, during a discussion of the Beveridge Report in the Cabinet Committee on Reconstruction Priorities, Herbert Morrison, then the home secretary and a former leader of the London County Council, declared that, because some hospital services required a wider area of control than the boundaries of local authorities, he had an open mind about how they should be organized.[15] In the autumn of 1945, however, Morrison, now lord president of the council and leader of the House of Commons, attacked Bevan's proposals in the Cabinet. He conceded that nationalization combined administrative convenience and technical efficiency but feared that, because of it, local government would

[12] John Pater, *The Making of the National Health Service* (London: King Edward's Hospital Fund, 1981), 178: "Drawing on his EHS experience and looking to the nationalization proposals of various kinds . . . Hawton suggested—and Bevan readily agreed—that the Gordian knot of the hospital service might be cut by taking over ownership of all of them but entrusting their administration to new *ad hoc* appointed voluntary bodies."

[13] Jameson described the nationalization of the voluntaries as part of the gradual development of consensus during the war: "It soon became clear to all that much of this was too good ever to lose," in "Replanning Britain's Health Services," *Canadian Journal of Public Health*, May 1946, 37: 173-181. His biographer stressed the same theme: Nevill M. Goodman, *Wilson Jameson: Architect of National Health* (London: George Allen and Unwin, 1970), 96, 195.

[14] "National Health Service Hospitals Scheme," August 1945. MH 80/29, PRO makes it clear that the ministry knew that what the government proposed to abolish was voluntary subscriptions rather than the power of the governors of voluntary hospitals. Moreover, it was clear that the proposal would cause "the biggest reduction yet made in the powers of local authorities." Contrary to Pater's interpretation, there is evidence that senior civil servants acted throughout August and September of 1945 as if the nationalization plan might be abandoned. The minister was reminded on several occasions that the old plans were "practically ready" and warned of "violent opposition" from local authorities if the decision were sustained. The first draft of the plan setting forth the new policy was not written until September 22, 1945, MH 80/34, PRO.

[15] August 17, 1943. CAB 87/13, PR (43) 49, PRO.

languish and Labour councillors would be divided. Moreover, the proposed regional boards and management committees would, he said, be free to set policy for which the central government would then have to pay.[16]

Prime Minister Clement Attlee understood that the dispute between Bevan and Morrison obscured their agreement on the fundamental issues of health policy. They agreed, he said, that the Exchequer should pay most of the costs of a National Health Service. Moreover, they knew that regional boards and hospital management committees would probably make the same decisions as the joint committees of voluntary and local authority officials proposed in 1944 and 1945.[17] Most important, like most Britons, and unlike their American counterparts, Bevan and Morrison were entirely comfortable with a dominant role for central government. Neither Morrison nor anyone else advocated local authority control of health services with the intensity that defenders of states' rights brought to similar debates in the United States.

Attlee and the Cabinet also knew that nationalizing the hospitals would not damage Labour among voters. The dismay of local councillors was balanced by enthusiasm about nationalization among leaders of the Trades Union Congress, who were hostile to voluntary hospitals.[18] Moreover, nationalization was unlikely to excite a broader public than the groups who were immediately affected by it. The general public wanted a free health service but, opinion polls indicated, with considerably less fervor than it wanted either new housing or full employment.[19] The complaints against nationalization by local authority leaders and the governors of small voluntary hospitals would probably be ignored as an administrative squabble. The predominant feeling in the Cabinet, Attlee summed up, was in favor of nationalization in order, as Bevan exulted in his moment of triumph, "to grasp an opportunity that comes but once in a generation."[20]

---

[16] "The Future of the Hospital Services," October 12, 1945, CAB 129/3 (04244), PRO.

[17] Cabinet Minutes, October 18, 1945, CAB 129/3, PRO.

[18] The TUC criticized the voluntaries in correspondence with the ministry in August 1945; endorsed Bevan's proposals in a meeting on January 8, 1946; and confirmed this endorsement in writing on May 6, 1946. MH 77/73, PRO.

[19] A.C.H. Smith, *Paper Voices: The Popular Press and Social Change, 1935-1965* (London: Chatto and Windus, 1975), 26, noted that a 1945 poll measuring priorities indicated that health services were a considerably less important issue of public concern than housing or employment and were regarded as part of social security in general.

[20] Note 17, above.

Attlee's judgment was confirmed by events. In the months between the Cabinet decision and the submission of the NHS bill to Parliament, in March 1946, the leading interest groups pledged to support the Government during confidential meetings at the ministry. In January 1946, for instance, the negotiating committee of the medical profession approved the overall design of the health service, though it urged that all local authority services, not just the hospitals, be transferred to the proposed regional boards.[21] The British Hospital Association and the organizations representing county and borough councillors agreed to support the Government's bill while pressing for modest changes in it. The chief executive of the BHA said that he approved of the Government's intention to finance voluntary hospitals. Bevan, conciliatory in victory, reassured him that the new hospital management committees would be self-governing bodies.[22] A few weeks later, when the civil servants met with officers of the County Councils Association, Lord Latham, now leader of the LCC, deplored nationalizing hospitals as an encroachment on local government but promised to support the Government's proposal if control of the voluntaries was also transferred to the Minister.[23]

Participants in the debate in the House of Commons on the NHS bill, in May 1946, expressed widely shared beliefs about policy to distribute the results of scientific medicine. Rejecting the advice of his civil servants, Bevan chose to emphasize the hospital service rather than comprehensive medical care in his opening speech.[24]

[21] Pater, *Making of the National Health Service*, Chapter 5, documents the negotiating committee's endorsement from the Royal College of Physicians Papers. Following its meeting with Bevan, the negotiating committee, "despite its opposition on some matters, decided to approve the idea of a national hospital service administered through executive regional bodies . . . in order to ensure the integration and correlation of the services they proposed that all of them should be administered by the regional bodies, though the general practitioners' contract would be with the local Executive Council."

[22] "NHS: Meeting with Representatives of Voluntary Hospitals," February 11, 1946, MH 80/34, PRO. Bevan told Sir Bernard Docker of the BHA at this meeting—without contradiction from Sir Bernard—that he knew that nationalization was "based largely on ideas provided by the voluntary hospitals themselves arising out of their study of the functional needs of a fully coordinated hospital service."

[23] Meetings of February 26, 27, March 14, 1946, with various local authority associations, MH 80/33, PRO. Latham's remark was made on February 27. Like the voluntary trustees and employees, the municipal councillors concerned with medical care were appointed to boards and committees in the NHS, and the staff of the local authority hospitals became NHS employees.

[24] "Suggested Contents of Second Reading Speech," n.d., MH 80/30 January-April

He argued that the cost of hospital care created financial anxiety, that hospitals were unevenly distributed, that they lacked a plan or system, that their facilities were inadequate, and that many were too small. In what became a famous remark, Bevan announced that he would "rather be kept alive in the efficient if cold altruism of a large hospital than to expire in a gush of warm sympathy in a small one."[25]

Bevan proclaimed his commitment to hierarchical regionalism. Hospitals were, he insisted, the "vertebrae" of the health system. They should be arrayed in regional units of a thousand beds, each unit linked with a medical school. Doctors must have an effective voice in managing these regional hierarchies; they deserved to participate fully in the administration of their own profession.[26]

Bevan combined belief in the centrality of hospitals and specialized doctors in medical care with faith in the wisdom of the common man. Because hierarchy and equity could be conflicting goals, doctors, Bevan insisted, must be subordinate to lay control. Moreover, patients—not general practitioners as the BMA had urged since the 1930s—had, he said, the ultimate responsibility to coordinate medical care. Users, Bevan told the House of Commons, would maintain continuity among the services of general practitioners, hospitals, and local authorities.[27] Bevan had little in common with Lister Hill, who had made the same points when he introduced debate on the hospital construction bill in the United States just a few months earlier. But they both tried to reconcile their commitment to hierarchy in organizing health services with a belief in the wisdom of ordinary citizens.

Most of the speakers in the debate on the NHS bill endorsed the Government's proposal to nationalize hospitals. A few Labour MPs

---

1946, PRO. The civil servants suggested that Bevan stress free access, personal doctors, comprehensive services, and the poor planning and distribution of hospitals. Their suggestion for advocacy of regional hierarchies was a cold statement of what Bevan chose to say warmly: patients need "admission to the *right* hospital for the particular complaint." *Cf.* Celia Davies, who writes that "official doctrine" in 1946 was not "hospital centered." "Hospital-Centered Health Care: Policies and Politics in the NHS," in P. Atkinson *et al.*, eds., *Prospects for the National Health* (London: Croom Helm, 1979), 67, 69.

[25] Hansard, *Parliamentary Debates*, House of Commons, 5th Series, vol. 422, April 30-May 1, 1941, cols. 43-44.

[26] *Ibid.*, cols. 46, 47, 50, 52.

[27] *Ibid.*, col. 30. Lord [Charles] Hill told Gordon McPherson in an interview, April 26, 1978, that "I asked Nye where was the coordination between the three parts [of the NHS] and he said that the patient was." (Courtesy of Professor Rudolf Klein.)

deplored the removal of hospitals from the control of local authorities. Several Conservatives and a few Liberals lamented the demise of voluntarism. Concluding for the Government, the parliamentary secretary to the Ministry of Health insisted that early treatment was the best method of prevention. Enthusiasts for voluntarism should remember, moreover, that the new boards and committees would have considerable independence and autonomy. Coordinating hospital and local authority services in the new regions would, he said, prevent much of the illness currently prevalent among the poor.[28]

The press and leading interest groups endorsed the Government's bill after the debate. Most of the national newspapers were enthusiastic about the proposed NHS. The Royal Colleges, after some well-publicized internal acrimony, voted to support the bill.[29] A prominent consultant reminded voluntary hospital governors, according to the *Manchester Guardian*, that because of public subsidy, real voluntarism had disappeared more than twenty years earlier.[30] The Society of Medical Officers of Health looked forward to a superb hospital service under the NHS and reminded the Government that MOHs were uniquely qualified to hold senior executive positions under the new regional boards.[31] In his presidential address to the society, in October 1946, Sir Allen Daley declared that the centrality of hospitals in the NHS was inevitable.[32]

Doctors' support for the NHS was obscured by the exaggerated statements of BMA leaders in the dispute over payment and working conditions for general practitioners during the two years be-

[28] Hansard, *Parliamentary Debates* note 26, cols. 70, 72, 146, 221-222.

[29] The acrimony was advertised in the House of Lords by Moran and Horder; Hansard, *Parliamentary Debates*, House of Lords, vol. 140, 16 April 1946, cols. 822ff. Support was presented to the public in a pamphlet prepared by a committee chaired by Moran: Consultant Services Committee, *A Consultant Service For the Nation* (London: Harrison and Sons, 1946). Reviewing volume II of Michael Foot's biography of Bevan, Lord Hill said he was surprised by Foot's revelation of the extent of Bevan's private consultations with the presidents of the Royal Colleges, claiming that he did not know about it in 1946-1948. Nevertheless, Hill admitted with some embarrassment that doctors were "slow to appreciate the wisdom of Bevan's courageous proposals for hospital unification." (Lord Hill of Luton, "Aneurin Bevan among the Doctors," *British Medical Journal*, November 24, 1973, ii: 469.)

[30] Professor Robert Plant, June 20, 1946, Clipping in JSM/MH138, PRO.

[31] "The Society and the National Health Services Bill," *Public Health*, May 1946, 59: 109-110. The LCC lost 32,000 employees in 98 institutions, which were divided among four regional boards and several teaching hospitals. It gained 4,843 employees in assorted public health and home health programs. LCC, *Report of the County Medical Officer for the Year 1947* (London: LCC, 1947).

[32] Sir Allen Daley, "One Hundred Years: A Retrospect and a Forecast," *Public Health*, November 1946, 60: 32.

tween the Parliamentary debate and the inception of the Service.[33] The vehemence of the BMA leaders was in part a response to Bevan's flamboyance and to the association's temporary isolation from the interest groups—the Royal Colleges and British Hospitals Association—with which it had been allied for a generation. Like the officers of the American Medical Association, BMA leaders and staff used symbols to capture the attention of the membership, which was absorbed in the details of medical practice. The leaders of the medical associations in both nations recognized that stating abstract principles in emotional language sustained doctors' interest in national issues and, perhaps more important, distracted them from conflicts of ideas and interests within the profession. In Britain as in the United States, leaders of medical associations had learned that their members preferred statements of implacable hostility to any policy or regulation affecting medical autonomy to bland reports about the interminable discussions and compromises of interest group politics.[34]

Despite their leaders' statements, most British doctors understood that the NHS was the result of a generation of consensus about health policy.[35] In 1947, the presidents of the Royal Colleges, mediated the practical issues in dispute between the BMA and the Government. Celebrating the inception of the NHS in 1948, Prime Minister Attlee, speaking on the BBC, declared that its goal was not merely to provide services for the sick but to make the nation

[33] In addition to the sources for medical support cited by Pater, the BMA made several public statements indicating that it supported most of the NHS. In April 1948, for instance, when the confrontation between Bevan and the BMA was allegedly at its critical point, a BMA pamphlet, *The Doctors and Mr. Bevan*, endorsed universal availability of services and worried about both a doctor shortage and the need for "more and better hospitals." Another pamphlet of about the same date, *The Right Patient in the Right Bed* (BMA, n.d.), worried about an "urgent need of" provision for long-term care, and called for action by the NHS. The BMA official historian correctly viewed the years 1946-1948 as a time of struggle over limited issues of GPs' autonomy, not over the central premises of NHS policy (Paul Vaughn, *Doctors' Commons: A Short History of the BMA* (London: Heinemann, 1959).

[34] Harry Eckstein, *Pressure Group Politics: The Case of the British Medical Association* (London: George Allen and Unwin, 1960), found the BMA more "restrained" than the AMA (71).

[35] The medical profession was growing in wealth and prestige. For instance, in 1948 the Medical Curriculum Committee of the BMA, in *The Training of a Doctor* (London: Butterworth and Co., 1948), expressed pride that applications to medical schools were running ten to one above prewar levels and that a survey indicated that more British parents wanted their children to become doctors than any other profession (10).

healthy. He had no reason to ask what evidence justified assuming that medical services would achieve this goal. The point was self-evident. The headline in the *Daily Herald* for the story reporting this speech summarized the history of health policy since Lloyd George introduced his insurance program thirty-five years earlier: "Attlee thanks the pioneers."[36]

The National Health Service Act and the Hill-Burton Act seem to have in common only their passage in 1946. The National Health Service promised to provide medical care that was, in the language of social policy, comprehensive, universal, and financed by tax revenue and social insurance. The Hill-Burton program, in sharp contrast, subsidized constructing and renovating hospitals, a task the British postponed. The two laws, moreover, were based on radically different conceptions of equity in medical care. The British made entitlement to care a fundamental right. The Americans were committed only to the more equitable distribution of facilities.

Nevertheless, the two laws translated similar beliefs into policy. The authors and managers of both the NHS and the Hill-Burton program assumed that medical care that applied the finding of science was the basis of policy to improve a nation's health and that hospitals were the central institutions of medical care. The NHS mandated that hospitals be organized in hierarchies within geographical regions; Hill-Burton decentralized the opportunity to regionalize in hierarchies to coalitions within the states. Both the NHS and Hill-Burton, that is, implemented a consensus that had emerged in each country since the beginning of the century.

THE ABDICATION OF LAY AUTHORITY IN BRITAIN, 1948-1951

By 1950, the Government established the limits of its willingness to dominate the allocation of resources within the National Health Service. British civil servants, like their counterparts in the United States Public Health Service, were eager to accommodate the interests of colleagues at other levels of government.[37] Officials of the Ministry of Health deferred to members of the new regional health boards and hospital management committees and encouraged their

---

[36] *Daily Herald*, July 5, 1948.

[37] R.G.S. Brown, *Reorganizing the National Health Service: A Case Study in Administrative Change* (Oxford: Basil Blackwell, 1979), 11; J.A.G. Griffith, *Central Departments and Local Authorities* (London: George Allen and Unwin, 1966), 462. For the United States Public Health Service, see Rufus E. Miles, Jr., *The Department of Health, Education and Welfare* (New York: Praeger, 1974), 168-219.

aspirations for more resources.[38] As the costs of the NHS grew beyond the Government's estimates, however, the Cabinet asked whether it was possible to limit the public's utilization of medical care.

The Ministry of Health encouraged the new regional boards to demand more resources, despite the austerity of postwar Britain. The ministry published ideal standards for services in order to emphasize the urgent need for growth. These standards described the proper number of medical and surgical beds as approximately 7.5 per 1,000 people, two-thirds higher than the ratio used by the hospital surveyors during the war and by the American authors of the Hill-Burton Act. Because of ambiguities in the document, moreover, contemporary calculations of ideal ratios ranged between 7 and 14 beds per 1,000.[39]

These standards could not be met without more resources. There were not enough qualified consultants in any specialty to staff the number of beds officials of the ministry considered to be desirable. New hospitals could not be built because housing had priority in the allocation of construction materials and labor. The standards set by the ministry, that is, encouraged doctors and members of regional boards and hospital committees to be dissatisfied about staffing and facilities.

[38] James Stirling Ross, *The National Health Service in Great Britain* (London: Oxford University Press, 1952), 161, declared that by policy the ministry gave the regional boards and hospital management committees "as much financial freedom . . . as general principles of Exchequer responsibility made possible." A committee of the Central Health Services Council, studied the results of passivity in 1950 and declared complacently that "it is unreasonable to look for perfect coordination," and that the problem of administration "was not created by" the NHS. The committee was chaired by F. Messer, a Labour M.P., and included Sir Henry Cohen, Sir Allen Daley, and Sir Ernest Rock Carling of the Nuffield Trust. Ministry of Health, Central Health Services Council, *Report on Cooperation Between Hospital, Local Authority and General Practitioner Services* (London: HMSO, 1952).

[39] Ministry of Health, *National Health Service: The Development of Consultant Services* (London: HMSO, 1950; first issued in mimeo in 1948); see page 2 for "tentative." For "ideal" see *Report of the Ministry of Health for the Year Ended March 31st 1949* (London: HMSO, 1950, Cmd 7910), 117. For a calculation of 7:1000, Nuffield Provincial Hospitals Trust, *Studies in the Functions and Design of Hospitals* (London: Oxford University Press, 1955), 150; for 6.5:1000, Vera Norris, "Role of Statistics in Regional Hospital Planning," *British Medical Journal*, January 19, 1952, i: 129; for 14:1000, George E. Godber, "Health Services, Past, Present and Future," *The Lancet*, July 5, 1958, 5. My calculation, from data in the document, was 7.5:1000. In 1958 Godber, who was a principal author of the document, regarded it as a "successful essay in general principles but not a reliable guide on details." George E. Godber, "The Physicians' Part in Hospital Planning," *British Medical Journal Supplement*, April 4, 1959, i: 115.

For the next decade, complaints of doctors and regional officials about inadequate numbers of consultants and hospital beds were amplified because operating experience was measured against the expectations created by the ministry between 1948 and 1950. They rarely mentioned the extensive renovations that were carried out within aging hospital walls in the first ten years of the NHS. Numerical standards were still used, as they had been in the wartime surveys of hospitals in Britain and the United States, as an index of deficit rather than as a tool to accommodate means to ends.

Moreover, officials of the ministry deferred to the judgments of individual doctors about how to allocate resources for all health services. They protected specialists' control of the division of labor in medical care as well as their freedom from interference by laymen or intrusive colleagues. An exception to this policy occurred in 1949, when Aneurin Bevan uncharacteristically declared that doctors were over-prescribing and patients were abusing drugs.[40] "Cascades of medicine," he proclaimed, were "pouring down British throats." But he soon accepted the advice of a committee of the Central Health Services Council that doctors should not be restricted from prescribing any drug they believed to be necessary for their patients.[41] At about the same time, the deputy chief medical officer told a group of doctors that the National Health Service was helpless to control what they prescribed. His chief, Sir John Charles, Jameson's successor and a former MOH of Birmingham, explained to the same audience that there was no need to establish priorities for allocating resources to curative and preventive services because the conflict between them had been resolved twenty years earlier, largely through the work of Sir George Newman.[42]

Not everyone was passive about the assumptions by which the NHS was administered. Sir Frederick Menzies, retired MOH of London, feared that the enormous cost of hospital services would force other medical services to be reduced.[43] A Cambridge radiologist warned in 1948 that, because of the freedom granted to doctors to control resources, national prosperity would suffer unless pa-

---

[40] Hansard, *Parliamentary Debates*, House of Commons, 5th Series, vol. 472, 14 March 1950, col. 924: "In November the Minister was saying that he shuddered to think of the cascades of medicine pouring down British throats."

[41] Central Health Services Council, *The Second Interim Report of the Joint Committee on Prescribing* (London: HMSO, 1950), 4.

[42] John Charles et al., "The Economic Aspect of Medical Care," *Journal of the Royal Institute of Public Health and Hygiene*, February 1951, 14: 66, 69.

[43] Letter to the Editor, "Hospital Costs," *British Medical Journal, Supplement*, December 11, 1948, ii: 220.

tients' access to medical services was limited by the standard of living.[44] Members of PEP complained that the regional boards and hospital management committees were spending money irresponsibly. Moreover, they said, doctors exercised disproportionate influence on hospital policy. But they still hesitated, as they had in 1937, to assert that the public interest transcended the preferences of doctors. Instead of reducing the number of doctors on the boards and committees, the authors of the PEP paper concluded, officials should enlarge them to include members of other health professions.[45]

Official permissiveness, the encouragement of a sense of deficit and the practical difficulty of predicting demand for services combined to create a financial crisis for the NHS in 1949 and 1950. In public, Bevan exhorted consumers to avoid doctors when they did not require one. Britain should not, he said, become a nation of hypochondriacs.[46] In the Cabinet, however, he demanded more money for the NHS and refused to reduce or restrict access to it. He dared his colleagues to take collective responsibility for diminishing the NHS, asking sarcastically which services they proposed should be withheld.[47] In the Spring of 1950, the chancellor of the exchequer, Sir Stafford Cripps, who insisted that he wanted to provide the best health services that the nation could afford, persuaded the Cabinet to impose a ceiling on the NHS budget. As a result, the ministry reluctantly imposed controls on what the boards and committees spent.

Officials of the ministry undercut these controls by insisting that costs were unpredictable because unmet need could not be estimated.[48] Moreover, for the first time the ministry contradicted the belief, first articulated by Lord Beveridge, that costs would stabilize as needs were met. Early diagnosis would increase utilization, Bevan and his officials insisted, even though the younger generation would be "imbued with the ideas of positive health."[49]

[44] Frangcon Roberts, "Where Are We Going," *British Medical Journal*, March 13, 1948, i: 485-489.

[45] Political and Economic Planning, "The Hospital Service, I, System of Management," *Planning*, September 26, 1949, 16: 94, 101, 107. PEP understood that the NHS was not a radical innovation: "It is a state service yet the managers are nearly all volunteers" (86).

[46] "Free Spectacles Rush Strips Bevan's Stocks," *News Chronicle*, October 8, 1948.

[47] "Circulated Cabinet Paper . . . Amendment to Last Cabinet," n.d. but appears to be April 1949, MH 79/622, PRO.

[48] Hansard, *Parliamentary Debates*, 14 March 1950, col. 938.

[49] *Report . . . for the year ending 31st March 1950* (London: HMSO, 1951, Cmd. 1951). The issues were confused by polemic. Regional hospital boards used increasing

Prime Minister Attlee created a Cabinet committee to review NHS expenditures. The committee was charged to recommend ways to limit expenditures at a time when the leaders of most medical interest groups, encouraged by officials, agreed that there was a serious shortage of consultants and beds and that existing facilities were rapidly becoming obsolete. The BMA had paused in its controversy with the Government in 1948 to assert that the nation needed more and better hospitals and twice as many doctors.[50] Lord Moran believed, as he recalled a decade later, that it was inevitable that the cost of medical progress must increase.[51] The professor of pathology at Charing Cross Hospital declared that hospitals needed more money because they had attained central importance in society as the leadership of the church began to fail.[52] A Socialist MOH asserted that medical care should be available for all patients who urgently needed it.[53]

Despite this consensus about the need to increase NHS expenditures, the Cabinet committee pressed Bevan to reduce costs. According to the committee, because the regional boards were expected to provide adequate services rather than to run hospitals as efficiently as possible, they tended to press their claims for funds without sufficiently scrutinizing them. Moreover, the boards usually chose the most costly alternatives. But the members of the Cabinet committee regarded the problem as one of financial, not of health, policy. They told Bevan to implement financial controls, not to reexamine his assumptions about entitlement to service.[54]

Despite what he said in public and in the Cabinet, Bevan was ambivalent about whether services should be limited in order to reduce

costs to accuse the ministry of over-centralization and to lobby for even greater decentralized (by which they meant RHB control over hospital management committees). Thus the Eleventh Report from the Select Committee on Estimates, *Regional Hospital Boards and Hospital Management Committees*, House of Commons, July 1951. *Reports, Committees*, Vi, 1950-51 (HMSO), made it appear as if too much bureaucracy was the cause of rising costs.

[50] On the BMA see above, note 33. In both countries, the myth that no appreciable hospital construction occurred during the 1920s and 1930s became accepted "fact" in these years. Wilson Jameson declared, "There has been comparatively little hospital building since 1919 in *Report of the Chief Medical Officer on the State of the Public Health for the Year Ended 31st December 1945* (London: HMSO, May 1947, Cmd 7119), 69.

[51] Lord Moran, "Lessons from the Past," National Health Service, Special Supplement, *British Medical Journal*, July 5, 1958, ii: 4.

[52] H.W.C. Vines, *Background to Hospital Planning* (London: Faber and Faber, 1952), 22.

[53] S. Leff, *The Health of the People* (London: Victor Gollancz, 1950), 245.

[54] Cabinet Committee on the National Health Service, May 10, 1950, CAB 134/518, PRO.

costs. At one meeting of the Cabinet committee, he insisted that hospital expenditures need not automatically increase. He hoped, he said, eventually to reduce costs by limiting hospital admissions to acute cases.[55] Four weeks later, however, he complained about shortages of beds and equipment and proposed to relieve them by granting authority to the boards to finance capital improvements through loans rather than from their annual operating budgets.[56] He did not resolve the contradiction between proposing one month to cap utilization and the next to increase investment in facilities. Four days later, he walked out of a meeting of the committee after Hugh Gaitskell, a rival for power in the party and now spokesman for the Exchequer, charged that, at its current rate of expenditure, the Ministry of Health would exceed its budget despite the ceiling. Medical care was different, Bevan asserted, from other areas of public policy. Hospitals and other health services were, he said, living organisms that should not be subject to conventional spending limits.[57]

After he persuaded Bevan to return to the meeting, Attlee proposed a compromise. Officials would force the members of the regional boards to reduce expenditures without telling them which services to curtail or eliminate. They would simply admonish board members to avoid drastic pruning of individual services.[58] Attlee's compromise removed competition for the resources that were allocated to medical care from the influence of general politics. What services were offered and used by whom, in what amounts, and with what effects, would henceforth be decided by experts in health affairs. Doctors would continue to determine priorities for expenditure because lay members of the boards deferred to them. The Cabinet would establish only the most general priorities, and officials of the ministry would agree with board members that too little money was available. The Government would watch while participants in health politics scrambled for resources.

Attlee's compromise appealed to Bevan and Gaitskell. Both of them were ambivalent about the propriety of withholding or rationing services. Although Gaitskell complained that consultants were overpaid relative to other British professionals, he agreed that spending for hospitals should increase. He later said that, in 1951,

---

[55] *Ibid.*, May 23, 1950.

[56] *Ibid.*, June 24, 1950, Memorandum by Minister of Health, "The Financing of Capital Expenditure Out of Loan."

[57] *Ibid.*, June 28, 1950. On Bevan walking out: Philip M. Williams, *Hugh Gaitskell* (London: Jonathan Cape, 1979), 214.

[58] Cabinet Committees, June 28, 1950.

he proposed to charge patients for false teeth and eyeglasses simply as measures of "financial discipline," not because he wanted to change the priorities of the NHS. Gaitskell had written in his diary that he "had always...said in the Cabinet and the Party meeting that if there were any more money available I would not have put it into the health services but done more for the pensioners." As chancellor, however, he permitted the NHS budget for 1951-1952 to exceed that of the previous year in order, he said, to avoid restrictions on hospitals.[59] Fundamental beliefs about medical care were too widely shared to be a proper subject for political rivalry.

Because Attlee's compromise was politically attractive, the Cabinet committee dismissed advice that the NHS's priorities should be changed. This advice and the evidence on which it was based were presented to the committee in July 1950 in a confidential report it had commissioned from Sir Cyril Jones, late of the Indian Civil Service. Because Jones lacked experience in health affairs, he mistakenly interpreted what he observed as a new mentality created by a free health service, rather than as the logical result of beliefs held by many doctors and officials since the early years of the century.[60]

The mentality Jones observed created what he described as almost total disregard of relative priorities at all levels of the NHS. Regional boards and hospital management committees were, he said, dominated by medical men who had a privileged position. The members of the boards and committees, he continued, submitted unreasonable budgets to officials who lacked adequate information about local events. Because national policy permitted consultants total freedom to prescribe, "in effect...the supply of appliances was accorded priority number one in the NHS." Consultants were, moreover, encouraged to be extravagant by the ministry's reiteration of ideal standards. Consultants in one region told Jones that official standards for medical staffing provided for at least five times the actual need. Jones was dismayed to find that hospitals' rates of occupancy were determined by doctors' behavior, that earmarking beds for each of the various specialties actually reduced their use, and that expanding the size of hospital staffs usually did not stimulate improvement in the care of patients.[61]

Jones's findings were set aside, although they were supported by

[59] Williams, *Gaitskell*, 262-266. Douglas Jay, *Change and Fortune: A Political Record* (London: Hutchinson, 1980), described the conflict between Bevan and Gaitskell, 197, 204.

[60] "Enquiry into the Financial Working of the Service," Sir Cyril Jones, Submitted June 29, 1950, 5, 9, 10, 30, 31, CAB 134/518, PRO.

[61] *Ibid.*

civil servants in the Cabinet Office and the Treasury. Officials of the Ministry of Health, who were annoyed by his attack on their passivity, insisted that the financial controls he recommended were already in place. Bevan agreed with Jones that doctors had too much influence in the hospital service and that they encouraged extravagant spending. But Bevan insisted that concessions to the medical profession had been required to launch the NHS. More important, Bevan insisted, medical care was too important to be governed by considerations of cost.[62] Bevan and the Cabinet were precluded by their shared beliefs from evaluating the benefits that were associated with particular costs. These benefits were, even Sir Cyril Jones finally agreed, entirely self-evident.[63]

Attlee's compromise, which made the temporary ceiling on NHS expenditures a permanent policy, was politically successful. The *Lancet* reported that consultants expressed very little anxiety that items eliminated from their budgets would not be restored. The major problem of the NHS, these doctors agreed, would be remedied by large infusions of capital.[64] Attlee's compromise even pleased Members of Parliament who had once been bitter antagonists. Charles Hill, who had been Bevan's principal opponent when he was secretary of the BMA and was now a conservative MP, declared that the NHS was properly organized and managed. In the same debate, Somerville Hastings, a founder of the Socialist Medical Association, said that Bevan had been wise to make concessions to doctors.[65] In 1948, Bevan had said what most people believed in a speech celebrating the inception of the NHS: "When we get into a hospital we must leave our differences outside."[66]

[62] Cabinet Committee, September 1950. Introducing discussion of the Jones Report (September 21, 1950, Minister of Health, Memorandum on the "Future of Regional Hospital Boards"), Bevan, in effect, set Jones's findings aside by ignoring his fundamental critique and claiming that his recommended administrative controls were already in place. Brian Abel-Smith and Richard Titmuss, who began an inquiry into the costs of the NHS in 1952, were not even told of the existence of the Jones report, according to a personal communication from Professor Abel-Smith.

[63] Jones assumed that the "legitimate grounds" for expenditure would be simply those that remained after the illegitimate ones were tested and removed (5).

[64] A Correspondent, "The Present State of the Hospitals," *The Lancet*, January 20, 1951, i: 165-167.

[65] Hansard, *Parliamentary Debates*, House of Commons, 5th Series, vol. 472, March 14, 1950, cols. 950, 1008.

[66] "First Day Rush to the Surgeries: But They Only Wanted to Sign On," *News Chronicle*, July 6, 1948. *Cf.* Paul L. Adams, "Health and the State: British and American Public Health Policies in the Depression and World War II" (unpublished D.S.W. dissertation, University of California, Berkeley, 1979), 384-386.

IX

A Policy for Growth:
The United States, 1946-1953

UNLIKE BRITAIN, where the NHS stimulated increased demand for health services in an austere economy, the United States prospered after the war. Demand for medical care was stimulated by health insurance underwritten by nonprofit or commercial organizations. The War Labor Board had encouraged employers to purchase health insurance in order to reward workers without paying inflationary wage increases. In the late 1940s, the federal courts sanctioned health insurance as a legitimate subject for collective bargaining. Moreover, health insurance as a fringe benefit received a federal subsidy because it was not counted as taxable income to either corporations or their employees.

Americans sought increasing amounts of medical care. In 1931, 48 percent of the population visited a doctor each year; by the early 1950s 72 percent did.[1] The average number of visits to doctors each year for each person almost doubled from the late 1920s to the mid-1950s.[2] Between 1945 and 1960 the number of admissions to community and teaching hospitals increased by 58 percent.[3] Between 1929 and 1959, consumer expenditures for medical care increased from 3.7¢ to 6¢ of every dollar earned.[4]

GROWTH AND HEALTH POLITICS

The proliferation of new technology to diagnose and treat illness stimulated public confidence in the effectiveness of medical care.

[1] Jacob J. Feldman, *The Dissemination of Health Information* (Chicago: Aldine, 1966), 32-22.

[2] Monroe Lerner and Odin W. Anderson, *Health Progress in the United States, 1900-1960* (Chicago: University of Chicago Press, 1963), 287.

[3] Joint Committee of the American Hospital Association and the Public Health Service, *Areawide Planning for Hospitals and Related Facilities*, PHS Pub. no. 85 (Washington, D.C.: USGPO, July 1961). The number of patient days increased at a lower rate, 36%, because the average length of stay declined from 9.1 to 7.8 days.

[4] Lerner and Anderson, *Health Progress*, 301. *Cf.* Louis S. Reed and Ruth S. Hanft, "National Health Expenditures, 1950-1964," *Social Security Bulletin*, January 1966, 29: 3-19.

Almost everyone knew from personal experience that X-rays and fluoroscopes gave doctors a privileged view inside the body and that antibiotics cured many infectious diseases. A contemporary historian said that it was no longer utopian to speculate about conquering tuberculosis, infantile paralysis, and cancer.[5] A statistician, summarizing the survey research conducted in the decade after the war, concluded that 84 percent of Americans believed that their chances of having good health were better than they would have been a century earlier.[6] This confidence in medical care also stimulated an unprecedented increase in the sale of proprietary drugs.[7]

Public confidence was, however, undercut by concern about the cost and quality of medical care. A survey conducted for the United Automobile Workers by Columbia University's Bureau of Applied Social Research, for example, found that the principal worry of auto workers was how to support their families and pay hospital and doctor bills.[8] As health insurance protected more people against paying the full cost of care, concern grew about its quality. A sociologist, reporting on attitudes toward medical care in a city of 350,000 people, found that respondents of every social class were distressed by a growing emphasis on technical medicine which took little account of personal relationships.[9]

[5] Eric F. Goldman, *The Crucial Decade and After* (New York, Vintage Books, 1960), 13-14.

[6] Feldman, *Dissemination*, 68-69: "There is some suggestive evidence that, not too long ago, doubts about the benefits of medical care were rather common. . . . That this is no longer the case is suggested by the responses to direct questioning on the subject, as well as by inference from the attitudes toward utilization."

[7] James Harvey Young, *The Medical Messiahs* (Princeton: Princeton University Press, 1967), 307. Stephen Strickland noted that a newspaper poll of readers in 1950 discovered that "items on medicine and health had a higher readership than any other category," *Politics, Science and Dread Disease*, (Cambridge: Harvard University Press, 1972), 125. E. L. Koos, in a study of the health and illness behavior of 514 families in upstate New York in the early 1950s found that in 17% of the households at least one person listened to radio health programs; 21% regularly read health columns in newspapers; 24% read magazine feature articles on health: *The Health of Regionville* (New York: Hafner, 1967 [1954], 116). *Cf.* Health Information Foundation, *All Their Powers* (New York; HIF, n.d., available in the Library of the College of Physicians of Philadelphia): "The stories in this booklet are adapted from five documentary programs broadcast jointly by HIF and the National Broadcasting Corporation over a network of 100 stations . . . subsequently re-broadcast over hundreds of local stations."

[8] Raymond Muntz, *Bargaining for Health: Labor Unions, Health Insurance and Medical Care* (Madison: University of Wisconsin Press, 1967), 49.

[9] E. L. Koos, "Metropolis: What City People Think of Their Medical Services," *American Journal of Public Health*, December 1955, 45: 1552, 1557.

Magazines and newspapers reported on the dangers of medical care while continuing to romanticize the achievements of doctors. The author of an article in the *Saturday Evening Post* complained that some hospital patients acquired worse ailments than they came in with.[10] Can we trust all our doctors, asked a physician writing in the *Ladies Home Journal*?[11] A spokesman for the AMA complained to *Time* that doctors often created a false illusion that medicine was an exact science and that they were infallible.[12] The editors of *Fortune* deplored what they called the geologically older level of medicine practiced in many rural areas, adding a new metaphor to the older ones of lag and gaps.[13]

These troublesome problems did not markedly reduce optimism about medicine. A doctor in Alabama, for instance, described in rural microcosm the impact of rising demand for care. By the late 1940s, J. Paul Jones was the only doctor in Camden, a town which, with surrounding farms, had about 9,000 inhabitants, 73 percent of whom were black. County officials applied for Hill-Burton funds to build a clinic after Jones agreed to pay the local share of costs from his personal savings. Jones hoped that the new clinic would reduce his work. Instead, his patients increased from thirty to almost seventy a day.[14]

Prominent doctors often applauded and reinforced public enthusiasm for medicine. In a public lecture in 1947, for example, the Homans Professor of Surgery at Harvard bragged that, as a result of scientific medicine, most disease could now be recognized and dealt with in early and remediable stages.[15] Ray Lyman Wilbur, who had chaired the Committee on the Costs of Medical Care almost twenty years earlier, said that he was pleased that the doctor was becoming a human engineer protecting persons against the hazards of life.[16] Surgeon General Thomas Parran said that public and voluntary ac-

[10] Steven M. Spencer, "The Hospitals Fight Their Toughest War," *Saturday Evening Post*, May 17, 1958, 230: 23-24.

[11] Dr. John T.T. Hundley, "Can We Trust *ALL* Our Doctors?" *Ladies Home Journal*, March 1953, 70: 53ff.

[12] "Dr. Superman," *Time*, January 31, 1955, 65: 14.

[13] "America and the Future: United States Medicine in Transition," *Fortune*, 1944, 30: 156-163 (quoted in Dean Clark, "Problems in the Distribution of Medical Care," *New England Journal of Medicine*, June 10, 1946, 234: 57).

[14] J. Paul Jones, "A Doctor Supplies a Community's Need," *GP*, June 1954, 9: 97-102.

[15] Edward D. Churchill, in Nathaniel W. Faxon, ed., *The Hospital in Contemporary Life* (Cambridge: Harvard University Press, 1949), 43.

[16] Edgar E. Robinson and Paul C. Edwards, eds., *The Memoirs of Ray Layman Wilbur* (Palo Alto: Stanford University Press, 1960), 622.

tion now brought the benefits of modern medicine to the smallest communities.[17] Most important, academic doctors, organized by Mary Lasker and her colleagues to promote increases in the budget of the National Institutes of Health, testified to Congress and the mass media about the triumphs of medical research.[18]

Growth became the goal of health policy. In 1951, a faculty member in preventive medicine at the University of Buffalo urged that hospitals and their personnel should be increased before considering the general problem of medical care for the whole population.[19] A study published by the Brookings Institution in 1952 concluded that health could be improved, as it had been for most of the century, without redistributing scarce resources. Hard choices could be postponed if federal and state governments subsidized an increasing supply of facilities and manpower, and thus of available medical care.[20] Moreover, growth in the supply of medical services was not controversial. A sociologist, for instance, found that because of Americans' unique regard for medical care, they were willing to purchase more of it.[21]

Several veterans of the battles about health policy in the 1930s now suggested that growth might be a means to distribute services more equitably. C. Rufus Rorem, a health planner, and Louis Reed, an economist, for example, endorsed private health insurance as an expedient alternative to the mandatory coverage advocated by other reformers.[22] Arthur Altmeyer, of the Social Security Board, recalled in his memoirs that by the late 1940s he advocated incremen-

[17] Thomas Parran, "Medical Services of the Future," *Yale Review*, March 1946, 35: 388-389.

[18] Strickland, *Politics, passim.*

[19] Milton Terris, "Medical Care for the Needy and Historically Needy," in *Annals of the American Academy of Political and Social Science*, January 1951, 273: 84-92.

[20] George W. Bachman, *Health Resources in the United States* (Washington, D.C.: The Brookings Institution, 1952), 3-4, 7-8.

[21] Odin W. Anderson, with Jacob J. Feldman, *Family Medical Costs and Voluntary Health Insurance: A Nationwide Survey* (New York: McGraw Hill, 1956), 81. For the intellectual history of growth as a substitute for redistribution, see Otis L. Graham, *Toward a Planned Society: From Roosevelt to Nixon* (New York: Oxford University Press, 1976), 93. For a similar analysis of the coalition supporting growth in the supply of health services see Paul Starr, *The Social Transformation of American Medicine* (New York: Basic Books, 1982), 335-347, 352-363.

[22] [Louis Reed] Federal Security Agency, *Blue Cross and Medical Service Plans* (Washington, D.C.: USPHS, 1947), 242. Odin Anderson, *Blue Cross Since 1929: Accountability and the Public Trust* (Cambridge: Ballinger, 1975) describes Rorem's role in promoting voluntary insurance.

tal growth in medical services as a better strategy than uncompromising commitment to national health insurance.[23]

A few economists complained that policy which merely promoted growth in the supply and consumption of services was inadequate. In 1950, for example, several scholars asserted at a meeting of the American Economic Association that the benefits of expenditures for medical care should be compared to the results of spending for other goods and services. The pursuit of good health, Herbert Klarman declared, was not an absolute goal. Spending more for medical care without evaluating results, he continued, could divert resources from other uses without providing any concomitant gain in consumer welfare. But Klarman hesitated. Medical care might be such an extraordinary commodity that it would be immoral to calculate supply and demand for it or to weigh its benefits against those derived from other goods and services. Need—not demand—was an acceptable standard for the allocation of medical care because Americans wanted to make good medical care available to everyone.[24] The growth of medical services might be desirable without regard to their cost.

Frank Dickinson, a professional economist employed by the AMA, urged Klarman and other colleagues to persist in applying to medicine the logic of their discipline. Medicine was not a unique commodity because it alone caused health to improve, he insisted. During World War II, for example, civilians were healthier because wages increased. Doctors were, Dickinson said, simply small businessmen. They should be subject to the forces of supply and demand in a free market.[25]

THE AMA AND THE TRUMAN HEALTH PROGRAM

Dickinson's reasoning pleased his employers. The AMA was now dominated by the large but diminishing number of doctors who were uncomfortable about the growth of specialism and hospital practice. What Morris Fishbein called, derisively, the grass roots

[23] Arthur J. Altmeyer, *The Formative Years of Social Security* (Madison: University of Wisconsin Press, 1966), 216-262.

[24] Herbert E. Klarman, "Requirements for Physicians," *American Economic Review Supplement*, May 1951, 41: 633-645; *cf.* Daniel M. Fox, *Economists and Health Care* (New York: Prodist, 1979), 25-26.

[25] Frank G. Dickinson, "Supply of Physician's Services," *Journal of the American Medical Association*, April 21, 1951, 145: 1263.

movement in organized medicine became powerful during the war.[26] Thousands of doctors, particularly those exempt from military service, were anxious about losing more patients, and therefore income and prestige, to specialists after the war. They were only partially mollified by the grudging creation of a Section on General Practice by the AMA House of Delegates in 1945.[27]

Fishbein was a victim of the tension created by this fragmentation within the profession. Intense, urban, Jewish, an insider in medical politics and a vivid personality in the mass media, he personified the fears of the doctors in the grass roots movement. He had been the principal spokesman for organized medicine for a quarter of a century. His columns were widely syndicated, Congressmen regarded him as an effective and entertaining witness, *Time* put him on its cover, and medical societies in every state invited him to speak. Beginning in 1944, however, Fishbein was regularly criticized by AMA officers and members of its House of Delegates for the inflamed rhetoric he used in public debate, a political style he shared with his detractors. In 1947, his enemies forced him to retire as editor and spokesman for the association. The "kingpin of American medicine has been toppled from his almost mythical heights," wrote the science editor of the Associated Press.[28]

In meetings with the AMA's officers and staff, though not in public, Fishbein displayed a more complicated view of medicine than the leadership of the association would tolerate. He simultaneously embraced science, specialism, and general practice. Shortly before he was ousted, for example, Fishbein criticized AMA officers for encouraging the Post Office to use Luke Fildes's painting of the early 1890s, *The Doctor*, on a stamp commemorating the association's centennial. Fishbein dismissed the painting, and its sentimental appeal to AMA members, because it did not depict modern scientific med-

[26] Morris Fishbein, *An Autobiography* (New York: Doubleday, 1969), 271.

[27] James G. Burrow, *AMA: Voice of American Medicine* (Baltimore: Johns Hopkins University Press, 1963), *passim*. Cf. Richard Harris, *A Sacred Trust* (New York: New American Library, 1966). Neither author noted the relationship between doctors' words about their plight and the evidence presented in William Weinfeld, *Income of Physicians, 1929-49* (Washington, D.C.: U.S. Department of Commerce, Office of Business Economics, 1950). Some doctors had economic reasons to worry about their status: those in the largest cities and the rural areas of the southeast. These were not, however, the same doctors who fired Fishbein, engaged Whitaker and Baxter, and led the AMA in its political battles. The only inferences are either that these leaders were cynical and manipulative or that they operated from beliefs that were at variance with their economic condition. I prefer the latter interpretation; Harris and Burrow the former.

[28] Fishbein, *Autobiography*, 313.

icine.[29] Fildes's doctor, he said, was not doing anything. Just before Fishbein was ousted, however, AMA officers hired two experts in conducting media political campaigns, Clem Whitaker and Leona Baxter, to promote its political program. Whitaker and Baxter welcomed the backward-looking symbolism of Fildes's painting. They distributed it as a poster, with a disingenuous caption urging the public to "Keep Politics Out of This Picture."[30]

The AMA officers apparently preferred the simplicity of this poster to the more complicated message of *Life's* cover story of 1948, "Country Doctor," by the photographer W. Eugene Smith. *Life's* doctor was not sentimental about isolated rural practice. He incorporated the technology of contemporary medicine into his work. Smith represented his subject's frustration in the final photograph in the story. Dr. Ciriani stares at the camera over an inert girl whose eye he could not save by emergency surgery in his office. The accompanying prose summarized his dilemma: "His income for covering a dozen fields is less than a city doctor makes by specializing in only one. But Ciriani is compensated by the affection of his neighbors . . . and by the fact that he is his own boss."[31]

A psychologist commissioned by the California Medical Association explained, after interviewing doctors across the nation, that many of them were upset. Most of his respondents told him they felt insecure because they believed they had lost community respect. Their twin self images of benefactor and breadwinner were in conflict, the psychologist reported. Doctors maintained their sense of power over patients, he said, but feared that it was being challenged by the public. They looked to the past as more desirable and opposed national health insurance, he concluded, because they were afraid of change.[32]

Many doctors found that their desire for a simpler professional

---

[29] *Ibid.*, 260.

[30] Burrow, *AMA, passim.* Leaders of the medical academic elite interpreted Whitaker and Baxter as a continuation of Fishbein's approach to politics. James Howard Means, for instance, saw the firing of Fishbein as mere "face-saving" as the AMA continued its by now traditional politics: *Doctors, People and Government* (Boston: Little, Brown, 1953), 150-156.

[31] Maitland Edey, ed., *Great Photographic Essays from Life* (Boston: New York Graphic Society, 1978). Editorial intent was revealed in Time-Life Books, *Documentary Photography* (New York: Time, Inc., 1972), 159: "An amputation, a birth and a death were part of the doctor's day; his selflessness is captured in every picture of the essay."

[32] Ernest Dichter, *A Psychological Study of the Doctor-Patient Relationship* (Sacramento: California Medical Association, 1950), 2, 4, 6, 10, 21-22.

life was consistent with the platform of the right wing of the Republican party. In the congressional elections of 1950, many doctors promoted right-wing candidates by dropping leaflets from airplanes, standing outside polling places, and writing to their patients on office stationery. The AMA even lobbied for foreign policy, supporting the Nationalist Chinese and Senator John Bricker's proposed constitutional amendment to limit the treaty-making powers of the president. It was not unusual for doctors as individuals to be political conservatives. It was, however, a departure for organized medicine to identify professional self-interest with a particular stance in general politics. The AMA now saw the struggle against international communism as an extension of doctors' opposition to socialized medicine. Doctors with different political opinions quit the association, which lost almost 25 percent of its members between 1946 and 1952. As the AMA became smaller, it ceased to reflect the diversity of political opinion among doctors.[33]

The AMA's political effectiveness was as much a result of the problems of the New Deal coalition as of the power of organized medicine. The Truman Administration was preoccupied with foreign affairs, war, and the economy. It was, one historian concluded, unwilling to press for domestic reform except to build a record against Republicans.[34] A study of the conservative coalition in Congress concluded that many Democratic congressmen were disinclined to support programs favoring low-income groups.[35] The

[33] "Transcript of First Meeting," January 14-15, 1952, "President's Commission on the Health Needs of the Nation," Box 16, Harry S. Truman Library, Independence, Missouri, recorded (57) that the now-disaffected Morris Fishbein told Dr. Howard Rusk that AMA membership had declined from 140,000 to 107,000 in the "past few years." The classic description of the AMA as a sinister, effective pressure group is David R. Hyde *et al.*, "The American Medical Association: Power, Purpose and Politics in Organized Medicine," *Yale Law Journal*, May 1954, 63: 938-1022. After describing how the AMA had been the major cause of the failure of reform, the authors asserted (1021) that "developments in medical technology and public demand for more medical care" would defeat the AMA; the triumph of group practice was "inevitable" because of the "advances" of modern science.

[34] Harvard Sitkoff in Richard S. Kirkendall ed., *The Truman Period as a Research Field: A Reappraisal* (Columbia: University of Missouri Press, 1974), 91, Elmer E. Cornwell, Jr., *Presidential Leadership of Public Opinion* (Bloomington; Indiana University Press, 1965), described, from primary sources, the lack of commitment (and therefore of staff work) behind the Truman health program (168-169, 240-241, 246-247). William Pemberton, *Bureaucratic Politics: Executive Reorganization During the Truman Administration* (Columbia: University of Missouri Press, 1979), described the failure of the Truman reorganization program, despite the President's commitment to it.

[35] David R. Mayhew, *Party Loyalty Among Congressmen* (Cambridge: Harvard Uni-

AMA was assisted by what another historian called a developing climate of distrust in which all innovations proposed by liberals or the left were regarded with suspicion.[36] Another study concluded that President Truman and congressional liberals mistakenly assumed that the public did not require their leadership in order to rise up against special interests.[37] Moreover, according to other historians, several powerful labor leaders, notably John L. Lewis of the United Mine Workers, preferred the health benefits they had negotiated to the Administration's program.[38]

Both the AMA and the press exaggerated the influence of doctor-to-patient propaganda on the defeat in 1950 of several congressional advocates of compulsory health insurance. Many Democratic incumbents lost their seats because of opposition to the way the Administration was conducting the Korean War. Moreover, in several states in which the AMA was active in senatorial campaigns, the Democratic party was split.[39] Senator Paul Douglas of Illinois,

---

versity Press, 1966), 165-168. Susan M. Hartmen, *Truman and the 80th Congress* (Columbia: University of Missouri Press, 1971), 211-213, described the divisions in Congress and the administration and Truman's reliance on advocacy rather than strategy to promote his program. Like Monte Poen, *Harry S. Truman vs. the Medical Lobby* (Columbia, Mo.: University of Missouri Press, 1979), Hartmen argued that "Truman's dogged advocacy" of health insurance, civil rights, and other programs "paved the way for acceptance of most of them two decades later." The "paving the way" school has not demonstrated that legislation has ever passed because a minority advocated it rather than because a majority coalition was formed.

[36] David B. Truman, *The Congressional Party: A Case Study* (New York: John Wiley and Sons, 1959), 22-23.

[37] Alonzo L. Hamby, *Beyond the New Deal: Harry S. Truman and American Liberalism* (New York: Columbia University Press, 1973), 327.

[38] Edward Berkowitz and Kim McQuaid, *Creating the Welfare State* (New York: Praeger Publishers, 1980), 137. Starr, *Social Transformation*, 280-289, in contrast to most recent authors, continues to emphasize the symbolic power of the AMA.

[39] "Columnist Drew Pearson reported that Democrats privately conceded that they lost Senator Elbert Thomas in Utah, Representative Eugene O'Sullivan in Nebraska and Representative Andy Biemiller in Wisconsin largely as a result of the doctor to patient propaganda." Stanley Kelley, *Professional Public Relations and Political Power* (Baltimore: The Johns Hopkins University Press, 1956), 104-105. *Cf.* Carey McWilliams, "Government by Whitaker and Baxter," *Nation*, April 14, 21, May 5, 1951, 172: 346-348, 366-369, 418-421. *Cf.* Richard Harris, *A Sacred Trust* (New York: New American Library, 1966), 53, who notes that many of the candidates the AMA claimed to have beaten in 1950 "lost for other reasons" and ascribed the "legend of invincibility that the AMA built up over the years" to 1939 "when the Wagner bill unexpectedly died in committee, because Franklin Roosevelt wanted it to," not because of the AMA. (26). Similarly, Theodore R. Marmor, *The Politics of Medicare* (Chicago: Aldine, 1970), challenged the *Yale Law Review* study and its advocates (53): "The AMA is thus pictured as the supreme legislative string puller. . . . Neglected in

for example, believed that Governor Adlai Stevenson, not Everett M. Dirksen and the AMA, cost the Senate majority leader, Scott Lucas, his seat.[40]

The AMA's tactics—lobbying, advertising, and selective campaign contributions—were unsuccessful when opposing interest groups mobilized their strength. Organizations of veterans, for example, regularly defeated the efforts of AMA lobbyists to prohibit the Veterans' Administration from treating patients whose disabilities were not a result of military service. On an average day in 1950, for instance, only 5,000 of the 40,000 patients in VA hospitals had service-connected ailments.[41]

Even though the extent of the AMA's political power was exaggerated, many politicians feared its criticism and its cash. The AMA was not solely responsible for defeating legislation and candidates it opposed, but its threats were taken seriously by most politicians. Throughout the 1950s, most elected officials tried to avoid confrontations with organized medicine. As a result, health policy could not be made, as most social policy was, by a series of compromises to balance the demands of competing interest groups. Consensus, not a majority, was necessary to make new health policy.

Public Investment in Improved Health

The power attributed to the AMA and its state and local affiliates obscured the emergence of a coalition advocating subsidies for biomedical research and medical education. In the late 1940s and early 1950s, a consensus about policy for research and education was articulated by public committees and commissions and then translated into federal and state appropriations. According to a report by the president's Scientific Research Board in 1946, for example, the conquest of disease should be second only to conquest of hunger as a priority for policy. The discovery of new and better ways to diagnose and treat disease was the most important area of

---

this stereotyped portrait is the distinction between results the AMA approves (or disapproves) and those they produce. The AMA has few resources for coercing individual congressmen to change their votes."

[40] Paul H. Douglas, *In the Fullness of Time* (New York: Harcourt Brace Jovanovich, 1972), 390, 562. Douglas recalled, however, that "legislators accepted the conclusion that the voters were opposed to all forms of health insurance and that they should avoid an open conflict with the AMA."

[41] Paul B. Magnuson, "Medical Care for Veterans," *Annals of the American Academy of Political and Social Science*, January 1951, 273: 81.

research, according to the board. Policy should be on the side of history, it said. The mystery of disease was yielding to scientific inquiry, even if some diseases still resisted the skills of science. During the war, scientists had produced phenomenal discoveries. This investment must be substantially increased, the board insisted.[42]

Medical education, the board continued, was a public responsibility because it was dependent on research. If research suffered, the standard of training for clinical practice would decline. The federal government should intervene in medical education because state governments were derelict. A quarter of the nation's twenty-eight state medical colleges, the board complained, spent absolutely no money for research. Moreover, only a few states had provided financial assistance to private medical schools. Medical science, communicated through education, would, the board said, lead inexorably to improved care.[43]

A National Health Assembly, convened by the Federal Security Agency in 1948, agreed that policy should create more hospitals, encourage research, and train additional health professionals in order to improve health. According to the authors of the official report of the assembly, everyone in attendance agreed that the hospital was the proper basis of health policy; the instrument, they wrote, for bringing medical science to the people, and the fountain of scientific knowledge and its application to medical practice. Moreover, they continued, the public's faith in medical research properly led to demand for more and better trained physicians and for more equitably distributed medical facilities.[44]

Although Oscar Ewing, the FSA administrator, advocated national health insurance, he told the assembly that increasing the supply of medical services should have higher priority than subsidizing access to them. Health policy should close what he called, in the metaphor first used by supporters of hospital construction, gaps between supply and demand. The absence of a systematic method

[42] The President's Scientific Research Board, *The Nation's Medical Research, Science and Public Policy: A Report to the President*, vol. 5 (Washington, D.C.: USGPO, 1947), 3-4. Cf. Strickland, *Politics*, passim.

[43] Strickland, *Politics*, 7, 15, 25, 34. *cf.* George W. Bachman and Lewis Meriam, *The Issue of Compulsory Health Insurance* (Washington, D.C.; The Brookings Institution, 1948; New York: The Arno Press, 1976). This study, prepared for the Subcommittee on Health of the Senate Committee on Labor and Public Welfare in 1947, argued that the nation lacked sufficient research capacity, hospitals, doctors, dentists, and nurses "to make a compulsory health system work."

[44] National Health Assembly, *America's Health* (New York: Harper and Brothers, 1949), 40, 169.

to finance health care was a grave handicap, Ewing insisted, but it was now more important to recognize that there was not enough medical manpower, not enough facilities, and not enough research.[45]

The most elaborate declaration that investing in the supply of medical care should be accorded priority in health policy was the report of the Commission on the Health Needs of the Nation appointed by President Truman in 1951. Like the PEP Health Group in Britain in the mid-1930s, the members and staff of PCHNN talked with representatives of every interest group in health affairs. Just as PEP ignored the Socialist Medical Association, President Truman did not appoint to the commission Oscar Ewing, the most vigorous advocate of national health insurance within his Administration. The commission's report, like PEP's, set a consensual agenda for health policy.

Maintaining health, the members of the commission agreed, should be everyone's first concern after food, clothing, and shelter. Health, they declared, had become possible only a few decades earlier, when medicine had entered its golden age as a result of advances in medical science. Physicians held the key to health, according to the commission. Health policy should, therefore, increase the number of doctors and other professionals, build more hospitals and, the commissioners insisted, "support any worthwhile research idea."[46]

Economic growth and voluntary action would solve the problems of organizing and distributing medical services, the commissioners insisted. The nation would, they said, prosper because people would live longer. As a result of this prosperity, no patient would need to be deprived of resources to benefit another. Medical services for everyone except the elderly and the poor, whose care should be subsidized by the federal government, could be paid for by voluntary purchases of insurance, the commissioners agreed.[47] Group practice was an efficient way to organize care, but it need not

[45] Oscar Ewing, *The Nation's Health: A Report to the President* (Washington D.C.: Federal Security Agency, 1948), 8, 10, 37-38. Surgeon General Parran, having learned to accommodate to power, now disagreed with his superior, Ewing, and retired. The Assembly, he said, was not "well-timed politically" since "favorable action" on comprehensive national health insurance "was not then to be expected." Bess Furman, *A Profile of the United States Public Health Service* (Washington, D.C.: USGPO, 1973), 459.

[46] The President's Commission on the Health Needs of the Nation, *Building America's Health*, 4 vols. (Washington, D.C.: USGPO, 1952), vol. I, 1, 3, 11, 20-21, 24, 42.

[47] *Ibid.*, 3, 13-14, 38.

be imposed since it would increase naturally, a member of one of the commission's study panels wrote, as an extension of the influence of the hospital.[48]

The report of the PCHNN evoked widespread support. Most of the general and professional press endorsed it. *Medical Economics* reported strong support for its conclusions among doctors, despite AMA opposition to federal insurance for the poor and the elderly and direct aid to medical education. Ignoring the AMA, the Academy of General Practice endorsed the entire report.[49] Opposition was muted. A dissenting report endorsing national health insurance, which was issued by a minority of the commission's members, received little attention.[50]

Michael Davis, nearing the end of his career, was distressed by the consensus expressed by the members of the PCHNN that health policy should be addressed from what he called the medical rather than the economic angle. He worried that the physicians on the PCHNN would endorse the separation of policy for what medical services the American people should have from policy for organizing and financing care. Education, construction, and research, Davis said, were merely means to the end of distributing medical care.[51] In 1950, he had broken with Albert and Mary Lasker and their colleagues in the research lobby over the same issue that distressed him in the report of the president's commission. The Laskers and their supporters believed that priority in health policy should be accorded to biomedical research and medical education. Davis retained his longstanding commitment to a comprehensive program of services financed by national health insurance.[52]

The findings and recommendations of the PCHNN were, however, consistent with what Davis had advocated for more than

[48] President's Commission on the Health Needs of the Nation, Study Panel on Regionalization, Miscellaneous File, draft dated September, 1952, 23, PCHNN Papers, Harry S. Truman Library, Independence, Missouri.

[49] Clippings reporting general and medical press opinion on the report are collected in the Michael M. Davis Papers, New York Academy of Medicine, 1-4; *Medical Economics* editorial support, February 1953 (n.p.).

[50] Anderson, *Uneasy Equilibrium*, 129, for minority report. The commission, eager to emphasize consensus, relegated the dissenters to volume IV, where the views of both I. S. Falk and Frank Dickinson appeared. The remarkable publicity the report engendered—front page in many papers, full text in the *New York Times*, for example—emphasized agreement among groups that had frequently been at odds

[51] Confidential Memorandum to Executive Committee of the Committee for the Nation's Health, October 20, 1952, Davis Papers I-4.

[52] Poen, *Harry S. Truman*, 177-178.

thirty years. Like Davis, the commissioners believed in the primacy of medical care in social policy. Like him, they believed that health policy should establish a hierarchy of services based on knowledge, and they assumed that health would improve as the result of the progress of medical science. In the end, Davis endorsed the recommendations of the PCHNN. Medical care, he and the commissioners agreed, was not an ordinary commodity. Any increase in the supply of care—whether directly by building hospitals and offering services or indirectly through subsidies for research and medical education—was desirable, even if the increase was, for a time, inequitably distributed.[53]

The assumptions that Davis shared with so many of his contemporaries were gradually translated into policy by the federal government and many of the states. With strong support from the media and in Congress, federal spending for biomedical research grew rapidly. The research budget for fiscal year 1951 was double what it had been the previous year. The number of National Institutes of Health increased from two in 1945 to eight in 1952. The research budget was reduced slightly in 1952, as a result of the Korean War, but began to increase again the next year.[54]

Bills to provide federal subsidy for medical education, however, failed in Congress in the early 1950s. Deans of private and public medical schools could not agree on the relationship between subsidy and enrollment. Moreover, unlike subsidies for research and hospitals, federal support for medical education was not yet disassociated from the liberals' health program. For instance, a bill to subsidize the operating budgets of medical schools was sponsored by Senator Murray of Montana and Representative Biemiller of Wisconsin, who were prominent advocates of national health insurance. Nevertheless, several prominent members of the congressional coalition that had created the Hill-Burton program supported their bill until it came into conflict with more compelling political goals, notably Robert Taft's desire to placate the AMA in his quest for the Republican presidential nomination in 1952 and the fears of southern senators that the bill would be amended to foster racial integration.[55]

[53] "The Financing of Medical Services," draft testimony by Michael M. Davis to the Commission on the Health Needs of the Nation, n.d., Davis Papers I-4. Davis returned to the mainstream of medical care reform in his final book, *Medical Care for Tomorrow* (New York: Harper and Brothers, 1955), 297. Progress, he said, would occur as a result of growth, even if the reformers goals were thwarted in the short run.

[54] Strickland, *Politics*, 84-87.

[55] *Ibid.*, 155, documents the data in this paragraph but interprets them quite differently.

States took the initiative to increase public support for medical education just as they did for higher education in general after the war. By 1952, ten states had appointed committees to plan new medical schools. A quarter of a billion dollars, most of it in state appropriations and capital from the sale of revenue bonds, was committed to new construction in almost every school.[56] Part of the impetus for state aid came from the federal government, notably from the G.I. Bill of Rights and from the health research and hospital construction programs, which required matching funds.

Training for medicine was linked to medical care in a way that made it different from higher education in other fields. Unlike the preparation for any other profession, medical education was inseparable from the organization of medical care. States subsidized medical education to implement policy for planning and building hospitals and redistributing doctors. As Alan Gregg, the director of medical science for the Rockefeller Foundation, wrote in *Scientific American* in 1951, the "cost of medical education was part of the cost of medical care."[57]

VARIETIES OF REGIONALISM

In the United States, as in Great Britain, almost everyone concerned with every aspect of health policy assumed that it was necessary to establish and improve regional hierarchies of hospitals and doctors. Philanthropic foundations sponsored hospital councils and university programs to promote orderly referral of patients, the rotation of house staff, and continuing professional education within regions. The President's Commission on the Health Needs of the Nation found that twenty-one states had regional programs supported by either public or philanthropic funds.[58] By 1955, as a result of a dec-

[56] Benjamin Fine, "Medical Colleges in Vast Expansion," *New York Times*, March 2, 1952. Ten new schools were established between 1945 and 1957: "The Future Need for Physicians," *Journal of Medical Education*, January 1957, 32: 47-48. A survey of state government activities appeared in Herman B. Wells, "State Support of Medical Education" *Journal of the Association of American Medical Colleges*, May 1947, 22: 155-159. Health professions education and hierarchical regionalism in patient care were explicitly linked in G.St.J. Perrott *et al.*, *Education for the Health Services*. A Report to the Temporary Commission on the Need for a State University (Albany, N.Y.: Williams Press, 1948), 116-120. The authors invoked both George Newman and USPHS Circular no. 292 (see above Chapters II and III) to support the conclusion of the report: "State financial assistance to education for the health professions . . . could go a long way toward bringing about the actual establishment of the regional health services concept on a large scale for the first time in this country" (145).

[57] Alan Gregg, "Doctors," *Scientific American*, September 1951, 185: 84.

[58] R. L. Puller to L. Breslow, June 10, 1952, PCHNN Papers, Box 2, Truman Library.

ade of indirect subsidy by the federal Veterans' Administration to schools that took responsibility for physicians working in nearby VA hospitals, fifty-eight medical schools had a financial stake in regional programs to treat veterans.[59]

Many leaders in the field of mental health also accepted the assumptions of hierarchical regionalism. Most states regionalized their public mental hospitals and clinics in the 1950s. Moreover, theorists of what was later called community mental health advocated establishing hierarchies that included voluntary institutions offering services at different levels of sophistication.[60]

Even in the early 1950s, there was fragmentary evidence that many doctors who supported the AMA on federal legislation would also support regionalizing hospital services. A striking example of medical support for regionalization occurred in Hunterdon County, New Jersey. In the late 1940s, prominent citizens in that county said that they wanted to focus the "spotlight of science" on rural medicine. After consulting an expert from the New York Academy of Medicine, these civic leaders invited the New York University School of Medicine to plan and operate a new hospital that would be staffed by salaried specialists appointed by the school. The New Jersey Medical Society opposed the proposal as a threat to fee-for-service practice and to the free choice of doctors by patients. The Hunterdon County Medical Society, in contrast, agreed to participate in the project if the hospital would be managed by an academic medical center. Although the Hunterdon project proved to be an isolated example of salaried specialty practice, it influenced other attempts to link a medical school with a small community hospital.[61]

Several strategies for regionalization competed for adherents in

[59] John A.D. Cooper, "Undergraduate Medical Education," in John Z. Bowers and Elizabeth F. Purcell, eds., *Advances in American Medicine: Essays at the Bicentennial* (New York: Josiah Macy, Jr., Foundation, 1976), 275.

[60] Joint Commission on Mental Illness and Health, *Action for Mental Health* (New York, Basic Books, 1961). The commission was established by the Mental Health Study Act of 1955; its report reviewed recent history and projected policy for the future. Pages 256-275 recommend a hierarchy of services, but do not use the word. In this hierarchy, state mental hospitals would become regional intensive treatment centers. But hierarchical regionalism in mental health was different in one major respect from its counterpart in general medicine: according to the Joint Commission, "the field (is) suffering from 'lack of' verifiable knowledge" (p. 190). Thus teaching hospitals were not central to hierarchies. *Cf.* United States Public Health Service, *Planning of Facilities for Mental Health Services*, PHS Publication no. 808. Washington, D.C.: USGPO, for regionalization and hierarchy.

[61] Ray E. Trussell, *One Approach to Rural Medical Care: The Story of the Hunterdon Medical Center* (Cambridge: Harvard University Press, 1955), 16, 28, and *passim.*

the 1940s and 1950s.[62] The most successful strategy emphasized the collegiality of doctors without regard to differences in their training and ability. The Bingham Associates Fund at the Tufts New England Medical Center, for instance, disseminated advice and promoted referrals instead of, like Hunterdon, decentralizing academic specialty practice. Both projects, however, restricted the roles of teaching hospitals and specialists and avoided the contentious issue of how to finance more equitable access to medical care. Scientific advances had created the problem of how to distribute knowledge, declared Samuel Proger, the medical director of the Bingham Associates Fund. Medical scientists, he continued, could solve the problem they created if they would "complement but not supplant the family doctor."[63] The purpose of the collegial strategy was described somewhat differently at a meeting of the panel on regionalization of the PCHNN. Frank Dickinson, chief economist for the AMA and a commissioner, asked if promoters of regionalization were accelerating the decline of general practice. An advocate of collegial regionalization replied that his goal was to strengthen the GP in his proper place in a hierarchy.[64]

Other experts believed that regional hierarchies of medical service should be organized systematically, instead of waiting for persuasion and education to bring about reform. John B. Grant, a doctor employed by the Rockefeller Foundation who was assigned to the staff of the PCHNN, was an eloquent advocate of this strategy. As a student at the Johns Hopkins University after World War I,

[62] Eli Ginzberg, *A Pattern for Hospital Care* (New York: Columbia University Press, 1949), 34-36, surveyed "recent patterns of affiliation" and found seven dominant types. The annual reports of the W. K. Kellogg Foundation and the Commonwealth Fund catalogue their investments in regional consortia. The most thoroughly documented of the Commonwealth Fund's projects was in and around Rochester, New York: Leonard S. Rosenfeld and Henry B. Makover, *The Rochester Regional Hospital Council* (Cambridge: Harvard University Press, 1956). The classic study justifying continuing professional education on a regional basis led by a medical school was Osler Peterson *et al.*, "An Analytical Study of North Carolina General Practice, 1953-54," *Journal of Medical Education*, December 1956, 31, Part 2: 1-165. The impact of these regional consortia should not be exaggerated. Reporting findings in the region of the Rochester demonstration, E. L. Koos, *The Health of Regionville* (New York: Hafner, 1967 [1954]), noted that "not one of the Regionville doctors enrolled" in the educational programs mounted by the hospital consortium (81, 156).

[63] Samuel Proger, "Distribution of Medical Care," *Journal of the American Medical Association*, March 25, 1944, 124: 823-826; "The Joseph H. Pratt Diagnostic Hospital," *New England Journal of Medicine*, May 11, 1939, 220: 771-779.

[64] Hearings, Study Panel on Regionalization, April 11, 1952, 1693-1694 PCHNN Papers, Box 1, Truman Library.

Grant had been inspired by Lord Dawson's plan for creating primary and secondary health centers. During a quarter-century of residence in China, India, and Western Europe, he strengthened his commitment to hierarchical regionalization, which he described as the "only way to bridge the existing gap between medical knowledge and its social use." In the United States, he believed, regional hierarchies could be organized by voluntary action if government would provide more incentives similar to those in the Hill-Burton program.[65] The best way to meet the need for health services, Grant advised the PCHNN, was to improve the organization of present resources rather than to make vast increases in their supply.[66]

Some systematic regionalizers wanted the dominant institutions in each area to be public health agencies rather than medical schools and teaching hospitals. One of them, for instance, told the PCHNN that medical schools should not have direct responsibility to provide services.[67] Very few people shared this point of view. Public health agencies had pioneered in the creation of districts and regions since the nineteenth century. But except for diagnostic laboratories, public health agencies did not establish hierarchies of service. Instead, they decentralized work in the interests of administrative efficiency.

Other advocates of regionalization who emphasized equity as well as reorganization linked local voluntarism with the national agenda of liberal medical care reformers. Frederick Mott and Milton Roemer, for instance, agreed with John Grant and the leaders of the Bingham Associates and Hunterdon projects that regionalization was the proper way to implement the scientific progress that originated in university medical centers. But regional planning should, they insisted, eventually lead to achieving the liberal reformers' goals of group practice and national health insurance.[68]

Although members of each of the interest groups in medicine and

---

[65] Conrad Seipp, ed., *Health Care for the Community: Selected Papers of Dr. John B. Grant* (Baltimore: Johns Hopkins University Press, 1963), xiii, 184, 171, 33.

[66] Study Panel on Regionalization, Miscellaneous Files, n.d., PCHNN Papers, Box 2, Truman Library.

[67] *Ibid.*, E. S. Rogers to L. Bareslow, August 7, 1952.

[68] Federick D. Mott and Milton I. Roemer, *Rural Health and Medical Care* (New York: McGraw Hill, 1948), 499, 531, 494. David A. Pearson, "The Concept of Regionalized Personal Health Services in the United States, 1920-1955," in Ernest W. Saward, ed., *The Regionalization of Personal Health Services* (New York: Prodist, 1976), argued, without evidence, that "coordination" was a deliberate conservative alternative to the social reformers advocacy of "patient care."

the hospital industry accepted hierarchy and regionalization as abstract goals, there was considerable resistance to implementing them. The medical staffs of individual hospitals insisted on controlling internships and residency programs in order to assert prestige, to avoid accountability to university doctors, and to make efficient use of low-cost medical labor. As specialized technology proliferated, doctors insisted that it be available where they practiced rather than in regional centers. Advances in radiology and intensive care, for instance, were devised and disseminated from teaching hospitals; medical demand soon made them ubiquitous.

Many full-time faculty members of medical schools, moreover, wanted to avoid regional service and teaching responsibilities. Although most faculty members agreed with Samuel Proger that medical schools ought to influence practice, the most powerful of them wanted to exert their influence by creating new knowledge through research and disseminating it by teaching residents.[69] Medical service should not be synonymous with medical education, concluded the authors of a report sponsored in 1951 by the AMA Council on Medical Education and Hospitals and the Association of American Medical Colleges.[70] Similarly, fewer than half of the deans who responded to a survey in 1951 believed that lack of money was the major barrier to extending the influence of medical schools through active regional programs.[71]

The implicit commitment to hierarchical regionalism in the Hill-Burton program was also compromised in practice. The regulations implementing the program required states to plan hospitals in hierarchies. But the regulations defined a base hospital broadly: as either a teaching hospital or any general hospital with at least two

[69] John E. Dietrick and Robert C. Berson, *Medical Schools in the United States at Mid-Century* (New York: McGraw Hill, 1953), 51. S. Proger, "The Bingham Program and Regionalization," April 1952, PCHNN Papers, Box 2, Truman Library. Robert F. Loeb, chairman of the Department of Medicine at Columbia University, College of Physicians and Surgeons, wrote in 1952: "My own philosophy of medical education and its aim, medical care, is . . . First, you retain basic medical education at the highest possible scientific level . . . , Second, you build up facilities in the community so it is possible for the physician, ultimately in group practice, to practice the highest type of medicine as taught in Medical Centers." Loeb to A. J. Warren, March 10, 1952, Rockefeller Foundation Archives, RG3 Series 900, Box 25, Folder 194, Rockefeller Archives Center, Tarrytown, New York.

[70] Dietrick and Berson, *Medical Schools*, 63.

[71] Surgeon General's Committee on Medical School Grants and Finances, *Report*, PHS Publication no. 53 (Washington, D.C.: USGPO, 1951), 37.

167

hundred beds and residency training programs in two or more specialties which served an area of 100,000 people.[72] In 1948, when Oscar Ewing announced his support for legislation linking regionalization with compulsory insurance, Surgeon General Parran advised him that it was not well timed politically.[73] In 1952, John Grant complained that Hill-Burton provided only a "pattern on paper" for regionalization.[74]

Despite the urgings of theorists of regionalization about the importance of prevention, moreover, in practice, diagnosis and therapy were always given priority. In the United States, as in England, regionalization became a means to organize personal health services. Most ordinary citizens seemed to agree that priority should be given to personal health services derived from scientific research. In Hunterdon County, for instance, voters soundly defeated a referendum to create a county health department that would have been housed at the new medical center, despite advice from doctors and planners that preventive and curative medicine should be linked.[75]

In the United States, as in Great Britain, there was consensus in the postwar years that treating illness and extending life should be accorded absolute priority in social policy. Neither public officials nor doctors nor ordinary citizens wanted to set explicit limits on how much medical care would be consumed or to reallocate scarce resources from personal services to preventive measures. Expenditures for personal health services were limited only by the ability of the citizens of each nation to pay for them, not by their willingness. Everyone agreed that the resources allocated to medical care were inadequate.

In the absence of explicit standards to regulate the consumption of personal health services, doctors' orders drove expenditures for medical care in both nations. What doctors decided to spend on each of their patients—paid for by voluntary insurance and by individuals in the United States and by the NHS in Britain—determined how the resources allocated to medical care would be spent.

---

[72] The regulations, originally issued in February 1947, were amended to liberalize the definition of base hospital on October 17, 1947. However, the Hill-Burton Act was amended in 1949 to authorize $1 million annually in grants for "improving hospital operations and quality of care through such methods as regional plans." Paul A. Lembke, "Regional Organization of Hospitals," *Annals of the American Academy of Political and Social Science*, January 1951, 273: 60.

[73] See above, note 45.

[74] See note 65, above.

[75] Trussel, *One Approach*, 100.

X

The Priorities of
the National Health Service:
Britain, 1951-1962

AFTER WORLD WAR II, demand for medical care increased in both Britain and the United States. More children were born in the 1950s than in any decade since the beginning of the century. Because mortality from infectious diseases and malnutrition continued to decline, more children survived to receive preventive care, to have accidents, and, in adolescence, to receive services associated with their sexuality. Because life expectancy increased, there was more chronic disease than ever before.[1]

Although health policy in both countries implemented the principles of hierarchical regionalism, there were important differences in how the medical services of each were organized. British general practitioners controlled their patients' access to specialists and hospitals. In the United States, in contrast, as the number of general practitioners declined, patients increasingly sought specialists' services themselves. Moreover, as a result of the annual ceiling on expenditures for the NHS, most British doctors allocated scarce medical resources by rationing them; that is, by adjusting demand to supply. In the United States, because financing was open-ended and there was a national commitment to growth in health services, doctors' decisions stimulated the creation of a supply of services to meet the demand for them. Moreover, the willingness of Blue Cross, Blue Shield, and insurance companies to pay for services without regard to doctors' credentials or the size and sophistication of hospitals impeded the creation of effective regional hierarchies.

The most important difference in health policy between Britain and the United States was its social purpose. In Britain, achieving equity of access to health services was the principal goal of policy, as it had been since the 1930s. Technological goals remained subordinate to social justice. Thus the British invested comparatively

---

[1] The most succinct source for these data is J. N. Morris, *Uses of Epidemiology* (Edinburgh: Churchill and Livingston, 1975), chapter I.

fewer resources in hospitals, research, and medical education than Americans did. In the United States in the 1950s, these priorities were reversed. In the politics of growth, technological goals took precedence over equity, which, it was then easy to assume, would improve as a result of disseminating knowledge through regional hierarchies.

The Centrality of Hospitals in British Health Policy

Throughout the 1950s, hospitals received the most attention and resources within the NHS, although they were never accorded as high a priority in Britain as they had in the United States. Hospitals were the subject of more questions and debates in the House of Commons during the decade than any other issue in health affairs.[2] Between 50 and 60 percent of the NHS operating budget each year was allocated to hospital and specialist services.[3] Although only a very small percentage of the NHS budget was spent on new capital projects in the 1950s, almost every hospital in Britain was extensively renovated during the decade.[4] The nation had developed an "appetite for hospitalization," a journalist wrote in 1962.[5] This ap-

[2] Calculated from the indices to Hansard, *Parliamentary Debates*.

[3] Calculated from Ministry of Health, *Annual Reports* (London: HMSO, annual).

[4] The best source for capital investment in the rehabilitation of old structures and for the incidence of new construction is Department of Health and Social Security, *Review of Health Capital: A Discussion Document on the Role of Capital in the Provision of Health Services* (London: DHSS, October, 1979), especially 80-83, which challenges the myth that hardly any construction occurred between 1948 and 1962. Jonathan Tross of DHSS made this document available, at the suggestion of Professor Walter Holland.

The dominance of the hospital sector in the 1950s may account for the peculiar history of medical manpower planning in Britain. In 1957, a report—the Willink Report—to the ministry recommended reducing admissions to medical schools because of a prospective sufficiency of general practitioners between 1960 and 1970. Ministry of Health, *Report of the Committee to Consider the Future Numbers of Medical Practitioners and the Appropriate Intake of Medical Students* (London: HMSO, 1957). The policy based on this recommendation was reversed a few years later. A later study suggested that the committee did not take proper account of the lure of the Hospital Service; in the first twenty years of the NHS the number of registrars and senior house officers increased four times, while the number of GPs declined. John R. Butler, J. M. Bevan, R. C. Taylor, *Family Doctors and Public Policy: A Study of Manpower Distribution* (London: Routledge and Kegan Paul, 1973), 11.

[5] Richard Findlater, "Doctors," *Twentieth Century*, Autumn 1962, 171: 4. *Cf.* Christopher Ham, *Policy Making in the National Health Service: A Case Study of the Leeds Regional Hospital Board* (London: Macmillan, 1981), 155: "the balance of power was weighted heavily in favor of teaching interests and acute services. These were the interests and services which were predominant in 1948, and they maintained their position."

petite was, however, tempered by other priorities both within and outside the NHS. British governments, for example, chose to spend more on housing than on hospitals. Similarly, the NHS consistently allocated more resources to general practitioners and home health services than individuals or third-party payers did in the United States.

The public's appetite for hospitalization grew, in part, because the press and, by the end of the decade, television became enthusiastic about events in hospitals. The popular press increased its coverage of medicine and science. News and feature stories about the NHS, which at first provided information about political controversies, costs, and wages, gradually changed to emphasize new drugs and surgical procedures. Newspapers increased their coverage of the technological and scientific triumphs of medicine. Papers aimed at audiences of every social class regularly published feature stories and editorials complaining that an inadequate supply of hospitals and equipment prevented people from attaining better health.

Coverage of the tenth anniversary of the NHS in 1958 exemplified this change in the press' perception of medical care. The editors of the *Daily Mail* praised the NHS but complained that the hospitals were at once a triumph and a disgrace.[6] Their colleagues at the *The News Chronicle* worried that most hospitals were out of date but also lamented the decline of the general practitioner.[7] The proprietors of the *News of the World* were more optimistic. In 1948, the paper had regarded political controversy about the NHS as more exciting than what health policy might achieve. On the tenth anniversary, however, the editors published Aneurin Bevan's reflections on advances in the science and art of healing and a story about conquering cancer.[8]

In the 1950s, British women's magazines also began to resemble their American counterparts in their appearance and fascination with medical care.[9] Columns offering medical advice were now written by male doctors rather than by nurses or lay women. The

---

[6] Wayne Minear, "How Sick is the Health Service," *Daily Mail*, July 1, 1958, 4.

[7] Tom Baistow, "Our Hospitals Are out of Date—That's the Hard Truth," *News Chronicle*, May 9, 1958, 4: "Doctors Decline," *ibid.*, July 3, 1958, 4.

[8] Aneurin Bevan, "What I Think of the Health Scheme Ten Years On," and Anonymous, "Step by Step Towards Conquering Cancer," *News of the World*, July 6, 1958, 8, 9.

[9] Cynthia L. White, *Women's Magazines: 1963-1968* (London: Michael Joseph, 1970), 140, 216; *cf.* Raymond Williams, *Communitas* (London: Penguin Books, 3rd ed., 1976), 50.

setting of romantic fiction about doctors gradually changed from rural practice to urban hospitals. *Woman's Own*, typically, promoted a serial as a moving drama of life in a general hospital.[10] The BMA's promotional magazine, *Family Doctor* was self-consciously a women's magazine, suggesting that all domesticity was related to medical care.[11]

Medical care was now displayed more frequently in films and on television. In 1947, a decade after it was promoted by *Life* and banned in Britain, the American documentary film "The Birth of a Baby" was finally licensed by the British Board of Film Censors.[12] Television was more receptive to American programming, including medical serials, than radio was. In 1958, the Ministry of Health suggested in its *Annual Report* that television could stimulate desirable public behavior. A serial about an emergency ward—which appeared in a women's magazine, then on television, and later as a feature film—would, according to ministry officials, promote blood donations.[13]

Most leaders of the medical profession were wary of the growing interest of the media in their affairs. In 1950, the BMA criticized the propaganda used by the American Cancer Society to raise funds.[14] When *Picture Post* devoted an issue to an unorthodox cancer cure, canceling all its advertising in deference to the seriousness of the subject, the *British Medical Journal* attacked it for being insensitive to the canons of science and for using photographs to suggest, falsely, that cures had occurred.[15] The *Lancet*, in contrast, praised *Picture Post* for weakening the taboo against talking about cancer.[16]

A controversy between doctors and the BBC occurred in 1958 over a series of ten television programs titled, "Your Life in Their Hands." The BMA objected to the series because it showed actual

---

[10] "Woman's Own Brings You Yet Another Moving Drama of Life in a General Hospital—Based on the Famous TV Series," *Woman's Own*, May 7, 1958, 32. Other magazines sampled included *Woman's Magazine, Woman's Weekly*, and *Woman's World*.

[11] *Family Doctor*, April and July 1951.

[12] "The Birth of a Baby," *The Lancet*, June 21, 1947, i: 877.

[13] *Report of the Ministry of Health . . . for the Year Ending 31st December 1958*, Part II, *On the State of the Public Health* (London: HMSO, Cmd. 871), 40.

[14] "How America Fights Cancer: Publicity and Research," *British Medical Journal*, July 20, 1950, ii: 212.

[15] "Picture Post Investigates a Treatment for Cancer," *Picture Post*, September 9, 1950, 48: 31-47; "A Secret Remedy for Cancer," *British Medical Journal*, September 16, 1950, ii: 663-664.

[16] "Publicity for Cancer," *The Lancet*, September 16, 1950, ii: 375.

surgery, which, its spokesman claimed, would make viewers anxious and would, moreover, make it difficult for doctors to persuade patients to think in terms of health rather than of disease. This criticism stimulated a debate in the House of Commons on the propriety of the series.[17]

The controversy revealed what the media regarded as important in medical care. BBC officials said that they wanted to inform viewers that modern medical attention was available all over the country. Modern medical attention meant hospital care to the BBC; eight of the ten programs were set in hospitals.[18]

The BMA's leaders did not attack the judgment of the BBC's producers about the central importance of hospitals. They objected to showing surgery to the public. These doctors questioned the BBC's taste, not its priorities.

After conducting a survey, the BBC assured the BMA that the programs had done no harm. According to the survey, the programs did not diminish the high respect in which viewers held GPs and made little difference to the high prestige of hospitals.[19]

Over the next few years, many members of the BMA became more comfortable with the images of doctors and medical care that the media preferred. In 1959, the BMA's official historian described his employers in terms of media stereotypes. They were, he wrote, a composite of the whitecoated unsleeping research worker, the steel-nerved surgeon, and the humane and kindly family doctor. Yet he also shared doctors' traditional distaste for this romantic image, which, he said, was the result of "glittering-eyed public fascination" with medicine.[20] The BMA soon abandoned such reservations about the media. Its *Journal*, for instance, endorsing a television film, described what it called the high drama of transplanting a kidney. The press and television, the *Journal's* editor continued, had become more responsible.[21] More accurately, the media, doctors, and probably the public, agreed about what was most significant and exciting in medicine.

[17] "Disease Education by the BBC," *British Medical Journal*, February 15, 1958, i: 388-389; same title, February 22, 1958, 449-450; news items on pages 456, 510, 592, 899 of the same volume.

[18] British Broadcasting Corporation, *Your Life in Their Hands: An Enquiry into the Effects of the Television Series Broadcast in the Spring of 1958* (London: BBC, November 1958), 10.

[19] *Ibid.*, 28, 29.

[20] Paul Vaughan, *Doctors' Commons: A Short History of the British Medical Association* (London: Heinemann, 1959), xvi.

[21] "The Sixties," *British Medical Journal*, October 27, 1962, ii: 1113.

Consensus and Dissent

By the mid-1950s, the National Health Service was an established institution. The Labour Government elected in 1945 had implemented, with only a few changes, a consensus that had begun to form before the war. Several members of the Conservative Government elected in 1951 had helped to plan the NHS as members of the wartime coalition government. MPs of all three major political parties served on regional boards and hospital management committees.

In 1953, when the Government appointed a committee of inquiry into the costs of the NHS, a few Labour MPs worried, as Aneurin Bevan told Parliament, that the Government wanted to "mutilate" the NHS.[22] The discussion in the Cabinet that preceded the appointment of the committee had created the possibility, for a few weeks, that fundamental dilemmas of health policy might be confronted. Like the Labour Government in 1950, however, the Conservative ministers decided to keep confidential their doubts about the most popular public service in the country.

In late January 1953, R. A. Butler, the chancellor of the exchequer, speaking with the concurrence of the minister of health, proposed to the Cabinet an inquiry into the costs of the National Health Service. Butler said that the cost of the NHS would most likely increase each year for the indefinite future. Some costs increased, he admitted, because prices did and because the NHS urgently needed new buildings, drugs, and equipment. But there were other, controllable, sources of rising costs, he said. Because doctors no longer needed to take account of their patients' financial position, many of them assumed, Butler insisted, that the "sky was the limit" in prescribing and in advising surgery. More important, he said, the NHS encouraged doctors to use standards of care that were too high for what Britain could afford to pay in a time of economic decline. According to Butler, doctors would have to offer patients "something less than the best—or less than doctors think is the best." But implementing such a policy was politically impossible. Neither doctors nor the public, he regretted, would accept lower standards of care in order to limit services and, most important, reduce the number of hospital beds. The only way to lower costs would be to per-

[22] Brian Abel-Smith and Richard M. Titmuss, *The Cost of the National Health Service* (Cambridge: Cambridge University Press, 1956), 3, quoting the Parliamentary debate.

suade people to give health policy lower priority; to "relate the present and prospective cost of the Health Service to the other claims on the national economy."[23]

The Cabinet rejected this strategy, either because its members feared giving a committee license to examine the priorities of economic and social policy or because they did not want to antagonize doctors and the public. Prime Minister Churchill instructed the chancellor and the minister of health to charge the committee solely to recommend how to manage the NHS more efficiently. Moreover, the Cabinet explicitly prohibited the committee from commenting on the expenditures of other branches of Government.[24]

The committee, which was chaired by a Cambridge economist, C. W. Guillebaud, reported in 1956 that both the policy and the administration of the NHS were satisfactory. There was, its members agreed, every reason to hope that the NHS would increase the health and life expectancy of the British people. But the demands on the Health Service would not decline relative to those on other social services as Lord Beveridge had predicted in 1942, the committee members concluded. Demand would increase as medical care became more effective. Because there was no objective and attainable standard of adequacy, a policy of providing an adequate health service could not have any precise meaning, the members said. Health policy should, as the committee believed education policy did, simply provide the best service possible within the limits of available resources.[25]

The costs of medical care could be established more precisely than standards of adequacy. The committee had commissioned a study of the cost of the NHS from Richard Titmuss and Brian Abel-Smith of the London School of Economics. Titmuss and Abel-Smith concluded that, contrary to what some of its critics charged, the NHS was not wastefully expensive. The proper measure of the cost of medical care was, they wrote, the percentage of the gross national product spent for the NHS. This measure focused attention on the behavior of the economy as a whole instead of on the cost

[23] "Proposed Enquiry Into the Cost of the National Health Service," Memorandum by the Chancellor of the Exchequer, 28 January 1953, CAB 129/58, C30 (53), 177-178, PRO.

[24] Minutes of Cabinet Meeting, 3 February 1953, 128/26, C6 (53), 74; "Enquiry . . . ," 129/59, C59 (53), 11 February, 1953; Cabinet Minutes, 12 February 1950, 120/26, C11 (53), 80, PRO.

[25] *Report of the Committee of Enquiry into the Cost of the National Health Service* (London: HMSO, 1956, Cmd. 9663), 49-50.

and effectiveness of choices made within the NHS. The civil servants at the Ministry of Health who assisted the Guillebaud committee and provided data to Titmuss and Abel-Smith ignored Cyril Jones's 1950 report to the Cabinet committee because it had offended them.[26] Moreover, Titmuss and Abel-Smith agreed with the committee that medical progress would be continuous. The work of the hospital as an "aspect of humanity," they said, could "not be assessed."[27]

The members of the committee used history to justify their belief that medical progress would continue. The great advances in medical knowledge in the recent past had originated in teaching centers and were then disseminated to less sophisticated institutions. Medicine would continue to advance in the same way in the future.[28] The austerity of the present, the committee implied, must be endured.

Most members of Parliament expressed satisfaction with the priorities of the NHS when they debated the Guillebaud report, even though the committee had not met the goal of recommending economies set for it by the Treasury and the Cabinet. The principal Labour speaker was a doctor, Edith Sumerskill, who asserted that because policy for medical care was derived from the exact sciences it should be debated without acrimony.[29] Many members, both Conservative and Labour, applauded the Government's recent decision to begin the first program of new hospital building since before the war. The minister of health said that he was pleased that the proportion of the average general practitioner's work devoted to preventive medicine was increasing each year.[30] Most of the MPs who spoke agreed with a Conservative who declared that the Guillebaud report confirmed his belief that the NHS must take priority among the social services.[31]

A few MPs criticized some aspects of NHS policy. One member worried that the public was losing respect for general practitioners.[32] Another criticized the drug industry for encouraging doctors

[26] Personal communications from Professor Abel-Smith and John Pater.

[27] Abel-Smith and Titmuss, *The Cost*, 35.

[28] *Report*, 75.

[29] Hansard, *Parliamentary Debates*, House of Commons, 5th Series, vol. 552, May 7, 1956, col. 811.

[30] *Ibid.*, cols. 847, 854, 870. Turton paraphrased and repeated Ian Macleod's announcement a year earlier of the "first programme . . . since before the war" (*ibid.*, vol. 536, col. 1903).

[31] *Ibid.*, col. 926.

[32] *Ibid.*, col. 939.

to overprescribe. But he agreed with the minister that building hospitals should have priority in new expenditures.[33] Sumerskill, who questioned whether more beds were needed, insisted, however, that new hospitals must be built.[34] Another MP suggested that hospitals be returned to the control of local authorities because hospital committees were being run by their medical staffs.[35] A spokesman for local authority interests criticized the Guillebaud committee for not paying enough attention to preventing illness. But after seven years of membership on a regional board, he was satisfied that the loss of power of local authorities had been a natural result of the way services must be organized. Local authorities, he added, even did a poor job of running the ambulance services.[36]

Similar criticisms had been made repeatedly since 1948 by a small number of doctors and officials who dissented from the consensus about the priorities of the NHS. The critics' most frequent subject was the priority given to expanding the hospital and specialist service. The MOH of the Borough of Smethwick, for instance, declared in his annual report for 1950 that policy should reduce demand for hospital care rather than supply beds to meet it.[37] A year later, Sir Allen Daley, now retired as chief medical officer of the LCC, regretted what he called his "exultation and optimism" of 1946.[38] The rising cost of curative services, Daley complained, threatened the national economy.[39] Similarly, a radiologist accused doctors and their

[33] *Ibid.*, cols. 911-912.

[34] *Ibid.*, col. 876.

[35] *Ibid.*, col. 906.

[36] *Ibid.*, cols. 895, 904.

[37] [Hugh Paul] *The Health of the Borough in 1949* (County Borough of Smethwick, 1950), 10, 29.

[38] Sir Allan Daley, "The British National Health Services: The First Three Years, A Critical Assessment," *American Journal of Public Health*, October 1952, 42: 1232-1245.

[39] "Whither the Public Health Service," Minutes of Meeting of Metropolitan Branch of the Society of Medical Officers of Health, *Public Health*, April 1951, 64: 134. Other MOHs were having second thoughts: "Cooperation in the National Health Service, Memorandum of Evidence Submitted by the Committee of the Central Health Services Council . . . to Report on Questions of Cooperation," *Public Health*, February 1951, 64: 75-76, presented evidence of friction between local authorities and regional boards and/or hospital management committees. W. G. Clark's presidential address to the SMOH, "Our Affinity," *Public Health*, November 1951, 65: 23-25, complained that the "Hospital Service has been given a priority which has placed it in the public eye at the pinnacle of the Health Service," A. Elliott, "Money, Manpower and the National Health Service," *Public Health*, January 1953, 66: 54-61, attacked Beveridge's assumption that utilization would decline and called for a "critical examination" to "determine what part of the national resources should be spent" on the NHS. Elliott spoke at a meeting of the Association of County MOHs.

allies among hospital administrators of becoming experts in creating demand for services. The paradox of medical care, he said, was that although medical progress was of immense benefit to individuals, according it priority in social policy caused the health status of the population as a whole to deteriorate.[40] Similarly, a journalist complained that the way hospitals were managed deprived doctors of incentives to economy. He regretted that doctors' subjective decisions determined the pattern of medical care.[41]

Only one member of the Guillebaud committee published reservations about the priority given to the hospital service in the NHS. Sir John Maude, the retired permanent secretary of the Ministry of Health, deplored the widespread belief that spectacular advances in medicine and surgery had diminished the importance that should be accorded to preventive medicine. He believed that prevention was deemphasized because local authorities did not control the hospitals.[42]

Unlike Sir John, most advocates of transferring hospitals to local authorities did not want to change the priorities of the NHS. Leaders of the Society of Medical Officers of Health, for example, told the Guillebaud committee that, if local authorities managed the hospitals, they could reduce the cost of care without diminishing its quality or quantity. These MOHs were not interested in Maude's argument that the priorities of the NHS were wrong. Their priority was campaigning against the de facto governance of hospitals by consultants.[43] In an editorial in their journal, they condemned the committee for defending how the NHS was organized and ignored Maude's reservation. Like most members of the Guillebaud committee, the leaders of the MOHs agreed that more care should be provided in larger and more effective hospitals.[44]

Critics of the priority accorded to hospitals and specialists in the NHS did not, however, advocate coherent alternative policies. For instance, the radiologist who wanted to eliminate free and comprehensive health services in order to reduce costs, also asserted that

[40] Frangcon Roberts, *The Cost of Health* (London: Turnstile Press, 1952), 77, 140.

[41] François Lafitte, "Financial Problems" in Institute of Public Administration, *The Health Services: Some of Their Practical Problems* (London: George Allen and Unwin, 1951), 110, 112, 115-116.

[42] Sir E. John Maude, "Reservations About the Structure of the NHS," *Report*, 279, 284, 274.

[43] Society of Medical Officers of Health, Committee on the Costs of the NHS, June 1953. Minutes. SMOH Papers, A25. Wellcome Unit for the History of Medicine, Oxford University.

[44] "The Guillebaud Committee," *Public Health*, March 1956, 69: 122-123.

there was a shortage of beds.[45] Sir Allen Daley criticized the NHS's priorities, but also gave the service uncriticial praise.[46] Similarly, when Daley welcomed Aneurin Bevan's 1954 conversion to the opinion that local authorities should run hospitals under contract to the ministry, he insisted that managers from local government would reduce the administrative costs of hospitals without changing their priority in the NHS.[47] Moreover, he agreed with Titmuss and Abel-Smith that the NHS's share of the nation's resources, not its priorities, was the major issue for public policy.[48] By the end of the decade, another critic of the priorities of the NHS was convinced that advancing prosperity would enable medical care to be improved without increasing taxes.[49]

Critics of NHS priorities lacked ways to predict the effects of alternative policies. In the decade after the war, however, research on the effectiveness of medical procedures and on the epidemiological consequences of particular services began to suggest to a small audience new ways to choose among competing claimants for resources. In the mid-1940s, the first professor of social medicine in Britain, John Ryle, had insisted, for example, that doctors could not justify the cost of their procedures using scientific methods. Expensive hospitals and clinics might continue to be built for generations, he said, as a result of enthusiasm rather than science.[50] In the next few years many doctors in universities and research institutions amplified Ryle's point. Clinical trials of streptomycin, conducted for

[45] Roberts, *Cost of Health*, 193, 163.

[46] Sir Allen Daley, "The Health of the Nation," *British Medical Journal*, June 9, 1951, i: 1284.

[47] Sir Allen Daley, "Easing the Transfer of Hospital Control to Local Authorities," *Municipal Journal*, August 9, 1954, 62: 792. Bevan had written "Local Government Management of the Hospitals is Best," *Municipal Journal*, March 12, 1954, 62: 544-545, advocating local authorities as contractors ("agency basis") for hospital service. He made it plain, however, that power should remain where he had helped to place it in 1946—with the doctors and the ministry. An editorial in the same issue of *Municipal Journal* (539) criticized Bevan for wanting to "retain full financial control in Whitehall." A week later an anonymous hospital financial officer, in "The Financial Implications of a Local Authority Service," *Municipal Journal*, March 19, 1954, 62: 603-604, made it even clearer that in Bevan's new proposal "effective control of the hospital service is centered in Whitehall." Daley, however, ignored these arguments.

[48] Sir Alan Daley's review appeared in *Bulletin of Hygiene*, October 1956, 31: 1052-1053.

[49] François Lafitte and John R. Squire, "Second Thoughts on the Willink Report," *The Lancet*, September 3, 1960, ii: 541.

[50] John A. Ryle, *Changing Disciplines: Lectures on the History, Method and Motives of Social Pathology* (London: Oxford University Press, 1948), 23-24, 106.

the Medical Research Council by a group led by A. Bradford Hill and published in 1948, demonstrated new methods of clinical research. More trials were conducted during the next decade.[51] Looking back on the brief history of clinical trials in 1959, the editor of a handbook on research methods concluded that, after World War II, it should no longer have been possible for clinicians to discuss the prognosis and treatment of any disease without supporting their words with numbers.[52]

Moreover, epidemiologists asked increasingly precise questions, which had implications for policy, about the effects of medical services on populations over time. A number of investigators in the 1950s, for instance, recovering a venerable theme in epidemiology, claimed that falling rates of deaths from infectious disease since the nineteenth century were caused by changes in nutrition, housing, sanitation, and real wages rather than by innovations in medical science and practice. A few epidemiologists began to investigate the unintended effects of accepted procedures. For example, Alice Stewart of Oxford discovered that diagnostic irradiation of children increased their risk of developing cancer.[53]

Epidemiologists were the leading skeptics within medicine about the effectiveness of medical care and the inevitability of progress. As J. N. Morris wrote in his influential textbook, *The Uses of Epidemiology*, first published in 1957, it was "absurd" to ask if health improved.[54] But few epidemiologists in the 1950s were explicit about the implications of their research for policy. John Brotherston, for example, then on the faculty of the London School of Hygiene and Tropical Medicine, circulated a memorandum to colleagues in 1952 in which he accused the NHS of providing care on the principle that anything was better than nothing. Decisions about the priorities of the NHS should, he urged, be made explicitly. The Government's annual ceiling on expenditures for the NHS could, he insisted, be an incentive to ensure that available money was used to best advantage. According to Brotherston, the assumption that all medical

---

[51] Austin Bradford Hill, "Medical Ethics and Controlled Trials," *British Medical Journal*, April 20, 1963, i: 1043-1049, reflected on the history of trials and described the importance of the trials he conducted for the Medical Research Council on the effect of streptomycin, 1946-1948.

[52] L. J. Witts, ed., *Medical Surveys and Clinical Trials: Some Methods and Applications of Group Research in Medicine* (London: Oxford University Press, 1959, 1964), 5.

[53] Alice Stewart, "A Recent Survey of Malignant Disease in Childhood; A Study of Fatal Irradiation," in J. Pemberton and H. Willard, *Recent Studies in Epidemiology* (Oxford: Blackwell, 1958), 13-17.

[54] J. N. Morris, *Uses of Epidemiology*, 7.

services were necessarily beneficial would not stand scrutiny.[55] A few years later, he attacked the Guillebaud committee for standing "hypnotized in front of the *status quo*."[56]

Somerville Hastings, consultant, MP, and leader of the Socialist Medical Association, tried to introduce epidemiology into political debate. The NHS, he told Parliament in 1954, had made curative medicine available to everyone.[57] But, he wrote in the *Lancet* in 1955, curative medicine did not take account of rapid changes in he incidence of disease. There was less infectious disease as a result of better methods of prevention and treatment, but mainly because overcrowding in city housing had declined. Epidemiological research, he said, made it doubtful whether more hospital beds were needed.

Hastings did not, however, change his commitment to hierarchical regionalism. He used epidemiology to reaffirm the need for what, since the 1930s, he had called consultation stations linked with parent hospitals. Because Hastings emphasized infectious rather than chronic disease, he defined prevention as case-finding and speedy referral within a hierarchy of institutions. He was satisfied with the priorities of NHS policy, attacking instead, as he had for a quarter of a century, inefficient small general hospitals.[58]

Advocates of higher priority for general practice made the most important challenge to the priorities of the NHS during its first decade. Several studies concluded that many GPs were severely overworked, lacked up-to-date knowledge, and practiced with obsolete equipment in inefficient settings. The number of medical students entering general practice was declining, some critics said, because of the prestige and financial rewards of hospital and specialty practice. Lord Horder, for example, asserted that basing the National Health Service on hospitals rather than general practitioners was a fundamental error.[59] A controversial report, published in the *Lancet*,

[55] J.H.F. Brotherston, "Medical Care Investigation in the Health Service," in J.O.F. Davies *et al.*, *Toward a Measure of Medical Care: Operational Research in the Health Services* (London: Oxford University Press for the Nuffield Provincial Hospitals Trust, 1962), 18, quoting a 1952 memorandum.

[56] *Ibid.*, 39.

[57] Hansard, *Parliamentary Debates*, House of Commons, 5th Series, vol. 527, 1954, col. 895.

[58] Somerville Hastings, "Do We Really Need More Hospital Beds?" *The Lancet*, December 10, 1955, ii: 1240-1241.

[59] Mervyn Horder, *The Little Genius: A Memoir of the First Lord Horder* (London: Duckworth, 1966), 99. Nevertheless, Horder believed that NHI should have been made universal and that "the organization of hospitals by regions" was second in importance only to universal coverage (97).

described the deficiencies of general practice. The author regretted that the future of general practice was being determined by people who gave priority to hospitals and specialists.[60] The *Lancet's* editors, who agreed with the findings of this report, identified two schools of thought in medicine, each of which they characterized with a metaphor: one school asserted that modern medicine dwelt in the hospitals; the other that the heart of medicine was general practice.[61]

Advocates of these two positions debated with each other throughout the 1950s and early 1960s. This conflict had, however, little influence on the allocation of resources within the NHS until the mid-1960s, when the Family Doctor Charter gave GPs new prominence, but hardly dominance, in the NHS. Sir George Godber, who was a dissident voice within the ministry in the 1950s, later recalled that the senior civil servants and the minister routinely rejected proposals he and a few allies made to allocate more resources to general practice. The most visible result of the efforts of Godber and his colleagues to improve the quality of general practice during the first decade of the NHS was a modest program of loans to stimulate the formation of medical groups.[62] In 1957, Godber irritated his superiors by making public his dissent in a speech published in the *Lancet*. Hospitals, Godber complained, were the most expensive, the most monumental, and too often the most lauded part of the health service.[63]

Officials of the Ministry of Health tried to reconcile the doubts of the NHS's critics with the reassuring conclusions of the Guillebaud Report. Surveying the first ten years of the NHS in 1958, for instance, officials claimed that its priorities had been correct. Critics who charged that the service was extravagant had, they said, been proved wrong by the Guillebaud committee. Increasing demand for care was, they were convinced, a result of medical skill and scientific advance, both of which enabled more people to survive to old age. The advocates of general practice had a point, however; family

[60] Joseph S. Collings, "General Practice in England Today: A Reconnaissance," *The Lancet*, March 25, 1950, i: 555-585.

[61] "The Collings Report," *The Lancet*, March 25, 1950, i, 547-549.

[62] Sir George Godber, personal communication.

[63] George E. Godber, "Health Services, Past, Present and Future," *The Lancet*, July 5, 1958, ii: 3. A speech given September 10, 1957. *Cf.* John Brotherston, "Government Viewpoint . . . ," in American College of Hospital Administrators, 21st Fellows Seminar on the British NHS, London, August 1967 (Chicago: ACHA, 1969), 134: The hospital "is the powerhouse and, particularly in our health service, it has been given a monopoly of power."

doctors should lead the clinical team in each community. In the battle for health, officials insisted, recalling the impetus given to hierarchical regionalism by two wars, hospitals would first bring "reinforcements" to the family doctor and then "constitute the last line of defense."[64]

Moreover, civil servants said, the NHS had restored preventive medicine to its proper role. The chief medical officer, Sir John Charles, insisted, for instance, that until 1929, medical officers of health had been content to practice prevention. Between 1929 and 1948, their attention had been deflected from prevention because they were forced to take responsibility for hospital services. The NHS permitted them to restore their attention to the preventive and welfare services.[65] Satisfaction with the past and optimism about the future justified complacency in the present.

A NEW POLICY FOR HOSPITALS

Although civil servants and their allies in the medical interest groups were complacent about the priorities of the NHS, they wanted more resources to act on them. As national prosperity increased in the late 1950s, they pressed the Government to allocate more funds to renovate and build hospitals. In the early years of the NHS, advocates of more resources for hospitals spoke of a backlog of unmet need, assuming that equilibrium would eventually be attained between supply and demand. By the end of the 1950s, however, investment in building and equipping hospitals was usually justified as the price society would always have to pay for medical progress. Rapid advances in medicine and surgery, a committee of the BMA that recommended more hospital construction declared in 1959, made it necessary to provide more funds.[66]

Unlike their counterparts in the United States, British proponents of building new hospitals emphasized replacement rather than shortage. Most British experts were convinced that the ratio of beds to population in most regions was adequate. Modernization, not growth, was the major theme of the groups pressing for new investment.

[64] *Report of the Ministry of Health . . . for the Year Ending 31st December 1958* (London: HMSO, 1959, Cmd. 806), vi.

[65] *Ibid.*, Part II, 133.

[66] A. Lawrence Abel and Walpole Lewin, "Report on Hospital Building," *British Medical Journal Supplement*, April 4, 1959, i: 109-114. This report was accepted as policy by the BMA Central Consultants and Specialists Committee.

The formulas used by British planners to project demand for hospital beds were, like those used in the United States, arithmetic statements of shared beliefs. But the beliefs were different in the two countries. Most American projections of the demand for beds were derived from hypothetical standards for the appropriate length of stay for leading causes of hospitalization. These standards were based on the opinions of leading clinicians. American planners, that is, wanted the medical elite to set standards for the less able doctors who also practiced in hospitals. Ideal standards would encourage doctors to behave more rationally in regional hierarchies. Moreover, in the United States, rigorous standards for length of stay provided useful criteria for cost reimbursement. Such standards, if enforced, could reduce the incentives for both doctors and hospitals to keep patients in hospitals in order to maximize their reimbursement from private health insurers.

British planners, in contrast, measured the demand for hospitalization by observing how elite doctors behaved rather than by asking their opinion. What was, they believed, was proper. Planners assumed that the judgments of consultants in each region when patients were referred to them provided adequate data with which to calculate appropriate demand for hospital services. This analysis of caseloads, although it was conceived only as a tool for planning, actually reinforced the authority accorded to consultants by policy and public opinion. Unlike the United States, where doctors with varying levels of training and skill had hospital privileges, in Britain, planners assumed, there was only one standard for each region.[67]

Using these behavioral standards, British planners concluded, beginning in the mid-1950s, that they could reduce their estimates of desirable bed-to-population ratios. While average lengths of stay for leading diagnoses had been lowered in the United States, they remained close to what they had been before the war in Britain. British consultants, it seemed, adjusted the demand for beds to the supply at any particular time. Beds were always filled; there was always a list of waiting patients. Caseload analysis, that is, demonstrated that the demand for hospital services had been brought into

[67] The most influential caseload studies in Britain were conducted in the early 1950s under the direction of Richard Llewelyn Davies and published as Nuffield Provincial Hospitals Trust, *Studies in the Functions and Design of Hospitals* (London: Oxford University Press, 1955). Other studies reinforced those of Llewelyn Davies; for example, A. Barr, "The Population Served by a Hospital Group," *The Lancet*, November 30, 1957, ii: 1105-1108.

equilibrium with existing resources.[68] British hospital planning formulas, Brian Abel-Smith observed in 1962, were subjective: planners multiplied the number of patients of each diagnosis whom practitioners wanted to send to the hospital by the average number of bed-days used.[69] As a result of this arithmetic, the beds required for acute care in 1960 seemed to be about half the number calculated on the basis of hypothetical standards, based in part on American models, in the wartime surveys and in the early years of the NHS.[70]

Britain, according to most experts, needed better beds rather than more of them; modernization not growth. Constructing new hospitals was justified because medical knowledge increased more rapidly than the sophistication of the facilities in which doctors practiced. In 1962, the Government published a plan for remedying the accumulated deficiencies in hospitals and building new ones. The Hospital Plan was published at a time of relative national prosperity, when the Government of Prime Minister Harold Macmillan was encouraging systematic planning in every sector of economic life.[71] In medical care, as in manufacturing, modernization meant replacing obsolete remnants of the past. In the words of the Hospital Plan, knowledge and experience would not stand still. The authors of the plan used the word "modern" six times in the first page and a half in order to emphasize the need for change.[72]

[68] J. F. Davies, "Commentary" [on Barr, note 67] in *ibid.*, 1108.

[69] Brian Abel-Smith, "Hospital Planning in Great Britain," *Hospitals*, May 1962, 36: 33. *Cf.* J.H.F. Brotherston, "The Use of the Hospital: Review of Research in the United Kingdom," *Medical Care*, January-March, October-December, 1963, 1: 142-150, 226-231, for a review and critique of hospital research in Britain in the 1950s. *Cf.* R. Kemp, "The Golden Bed," *The Lancet*, November 14, 1964, ii: 1025: "What is clear from the figures is that the greater the number of beds the longer the patients stay in them."

[70] Gordon Forsyth, R. Glynn Thomas, S. P. Jones, "Planning in Practice: A Half Term Report," in Gordon McLachlan, ed., *Problems and Progress in Medical Care*, 4th series (London: Oxford University Press, 1970), 3, 4.

[71] Samuel H. Beer, *The British Political System* (New York: Random House, 1974), 71ff.; and *Britain Against Itself: The Political Contradictions of Collectivism* (New York: W. W. Norton, 1982), 122, on the emphasis on modernization in the Macmillan government.

[72] Ministry of Health, *A Hospital Plan for England and Wales* (London: HMSO, 1962, Cmnd. 1604), iii, i. *Cf.* David E. Allen, *Hospital Planning: The Development of the 1962 Hospital Plan* (London: Pitman Medical, 1979), 142, 162, for a different interpretation. *Cf.* Martin J. Wiener, *British Culture and the Decline of the Industrial Spirit 1850-1950* (Cambridge: Cambridge University Press, 1981), 162. When the plan was revised four years later, the integration of hospital with preventive and community service was a more important theme than modernization: Ministry of Health, NHS, *The Hos-*

The minister of health who presented the Hospital Plan to Parliament, Enoch Powell, doubted whether the NHS's priorities were correct. He told the Royal Society of Medicine that NHS policy was a mere bundle of public expenditures that were not even made as a result of arbitrary decisions.[73] Powell came close to criticizing the way the NHS had allocated resources since 1950, the process by which doctors', and particularly consultants', judgments determined how funds were spent under a ceiling set by the Government. But Powell, for once, did not complete his argument. He agreed with the medical profession and, it seemed, with the public that, in the words of a joint committee of the BMA and the Royal Colleges, "expansion of the hospital services with properly planned modern hospitals was long overdue."[74]

The belief that hospitals should be arrayed in hierarchies in order to create and disseminate medical knowledge was still the basis of consensus about British health policy. Presenting the Hospital Plan to Parliament, Powell declared that new British hospitals must be the equal of any in the world. He envisioned replacing almost half the hospitals in the country and completing the work of regional integration that had begun two decades earlier.[75] Replying for Labour, Kenneth Robinson agreed with Powell, although he complained that the Hospital Plan was a decade too late. Robinson, echoing Bevan in 1946, defended the priority accorded to hospital services: "There are those who believe that in concentrating on the hospitals the Minister of Health has got his priorities wrong," he said. "I venture to disagree with them."[76]

The Hospital Plan was the culmination of half a century of the history of health policy in Britain. There was little reason to doubt the effectiveness of the medical work performed in hospitals. Lord Horder had missed the point when he condemned politicians and doctors for making hospitals what he called the "apotheosis" of medical care. The centrality of hospitals in regional hierarchies of practitioners and institutions was taken for granted as the basis of British health policy. The relative priority of various levels of these

---

pital Building Programme: A Revision of the Hospital Plan for England and Wales (London: HMSO, 1966, Cmd. 3000).

[73] Enoch Powell, "Squaring the Circle," Twentieth Century, Autumn 1962, 171: 79.

[74] [Sir Arthur Porritt et al.], A Review of the Medical Services in Great Britain (London: Social Assay, 1962), 98.

[75] Hansard, Parliamentary Debates, House of Commons, 5th Series, vol. 661, col. 153, 160, 76, 44.

[76] Ibid., col. 44.

hierarchies would change in the two decades after 1962. Moreover, the priority accorded to hospitals in Britain, in contrast to the United States, was tempered by a commitment to maintaining and increasing equity of access to medical care. But the fundamental assumption that the National Health Service should be organized in orderly regional hierarchies remained unshaken and, even in the 1980s, largely unchallenged.

XI

A Triumphant Coalition:
The United States, 1953-1965

A COMMISSION appointed by Harry S. Truman had recommended a comprehensive health policy just before Dwight D. Eisenhower became president. There was substantial support for some of the commission's proposals for more hospital construction, increased biomedical research, regional hospital planning and coordination, and subsidized medical care for the poor and the disabled. Other proposals were controversial, especially grants to medical schools for education and a federal program of medical care for the elderly.

During the next dozen years, the commission's recommendations became national policy. By the end of Lyndon Johnson's administration in 1969, federal legislation had been enacted to subsidize medical schools, stimulate comprehensive health planning in states and regions, disseminate new biomedical technology from regional medical centers, and, most important, pay for medical care for the elderly and most of the poor.

BUILDING STATE AND LOCAL ALLIANCES
FOR MEDICAL EDUCATION

The coalition that had created the Hill-Burton program to construct hospitals expanded its agenda. Local coalitions were organized in almost every state in the 1950s to obtain public subsidies to assist the growth of medical education and hospitals. The success of a national coalition for health policy in the 1960s was the result of events in cities and states in the preceding decade. The most prominent members of these coalitions were leaders of state and county medical societies, trustees of large hospitals, industrialists, and labor leaders. They were supported by business, banking, and union leaders who had a self-interest in constructing schools and hospitals and supplying them with goods and services and by elected officials who were delighted to support popular programs and attract federal matching funds.[1] The members of each of these groups had dif-

[1] Vernon W. Lippard and Elizabeth F. Purcell, *Case Histories of Ten New Medical*

ferent political and economic interests. But they agreed, in general, on the content of policy to increase the supply of medical services and to subsidize demand for them.

Many influential Americans held similar beliefs about policy for economic growth and for medical care. Just as affluence would be increased by more investment in productive enterprises, they assumed, health would improve as a result of more hospital construction, research, medical education, and incentives to stimulate the growth of private health insurance. Only the poor and perhaps the elderly required special consideration.[2]

Many people agreed that supplying more medical care would satisfy demand for it in a prosperous society. At the end of the decade, Melvin Laird, a leading Republican congressman, stated the consensus as an epigram "Medical research is the best kind of health insurance."[3] Only the persistent advocates of national health insurance—who were the counterparts in health affairs of the economists who worried about structural unemployment and the impact of automation on the economy—complained that this trickle-down theory, as it was labeled by its enemies, would not remedy the inequitable distribution of medical services.

Doctors were the most influential advocates of the growth of medical schools and hospitals. Vernon Lippard, a doctor who helped to plan several new schools, recalled that medical societies often mobilized other groups to press state legislatures to establish new schools and support existing ones.[4] Many community doctors still feared that medical schools wanted to dominate the way medicine was practiced and to control community hospitals.[5] Other doctors, however, wanted the prestige and personal satisfaction of membership in a medical faculty. As the leaders of the postwar grass roots movement in organized medicine retired, specialists were more frequently elected to offices in county and state medical

---

Schools (New York: Josiah Macy, Jr., Foundation, 1972); cf. Centre for Educational Research and Innovation, *Health, Higher Education and the Community: Towards a Regional Health University* (Paris: OECD, 1977).

[2] James T. Patterson, *America's Struggle Against Poverty, 1900-1980* (Cambridge: Harvard University Press, 1981), 78-96.

[3] Stephen P. Strickland, *Politics, Science and Dread Disease* (Cambridge: Harvard University Press, 1972), 213.

[4] Vernon W. Lippard, *A Half-Century of Medical Education* (New York: Josiah Macy, Jr., Foundation, 1974), 72, 117.

[5] Stewart G. Wolf, Jr., and Ward Darley, *Medical Education and Practice: Relationships and Responsibilities in a Changing Society, Journal of Medical Education* (Part II, January 1965), v.

societies. Moreover, national and state societies of specialists were taking independent political action. The new leaders' education, their training in hospital residencies, their experience in wartime military hierarchies and, perhaps most important, their thriving practices—often group practices—made them expansive about the future.

The surge in public spending for medical education occurred at a time when it was sought by fewer and less qualified students. The ratio of applicants to places in the entering classes of medical schools declined in the 1950s. In 1958, the ratio was lower than it had been in the depression year of 1935. In 1953, the schools accepted 46 percent of all applicants; in 1961, 59 percent. Some schools, particularly those which restricted their enrollment to state residents, frequently did not fill their classes. Moreover, the quality of applicants, as measured by their grades and test scores, declined throughout the decade.[6]

Public financing of medical education increased in the 1950s as a result of both federal incentives and state policy for higher education and health. Federal grants for research and research training, and later for constructing facilities for research, supplemented state appropriations for education and patient care. Direct support for medical schools by states and cities increased more than 400 percent between 1948 and 1958. During the 1950s, medical schools raised matching funds from local appropriations or philanthropy for 126 projects financed by Hill-Burton grants in hospitals they owned or controlled. The number of faculty members in clinical disciplines who were considered to be full-time by their schools doubled from 3,500 in 1950 to 7,000 in 1960, mainly as a result of income from public sources.[7]

[6] John A.D. Cooper, "Undergraduate Medical Education," in John T. Bowers and Elizabeth F. Purcell, eds., *American Medicine: Essays at the Bicentennial* (New York: Josiah Macy, Jr., Foundation, 1976); Lippard; "Physician Supply and the Talent Pool: A National Problem," *Journal of Medical Education*, June 1962, 37: 618-619. The Surgeon General's Consulting Group, on Medical Education, *Physicians for a Growing America*, USPHS Publication no. 709 (Washington: USGPO, October 1959, 14), reported that "some medical school deans even now report increasing difficulties in filling their first year classes with acceptable students," and noted that the ratio of applicants to acceptances was 1.8 to 1 in 1958 and 1.9 to 1 in 1935. The total number of medical school graduates increased, however. Rashi Fein, *The Doctor Shortage* (Washington, D.C.: The Brookings Institution, 1967), 80, noted that "In 1966 American medical schools graduated 36% more physicians than they did in 1950 and 7% more than in 1960."

[7] Surgeon General's Consulting Group, *Physicians*, 37-49; Cooper, "Undergraduate Medical Education," 289, 296-297. *Cf.* Rosemary Stevens, *American Medicine and the Public Interest* (New Haven: Yale University Press, 1971), *passim.*

State governments were mainly responsible for the growth of medical education in the 1950s. State spending for medical schools was part of a general increase in public expenditure for higher education. Contractors and leaders of unions in the building trades, for example, lobbied for all subsidized construction rather than for medical schools and hospitals in particular. Each state, however, regarded its subsidies for medical education as part of its policy for health as well as for higher education.

Because health and higher education policy converged, states linked funding for medical education to regional planning for services. Nine new state university teaching hospitals opened during the decade. New state-supported schools opened in California, Florida, the state of Washington, and Puerto Rico. In New York state, the government assumed responsibility for two private medical schools; in Texas for one. Plans initiated or encouraged by state health and higher education officials in the 1950s led to the opening of fifteen new schools in the next decade.[8]

Name-inflation symbolized the convergence of health and higher education policy. All over the nation, hospital trustees, joining their own aspirations for higher status of those of their medical staffs, renamed their institutions "medical centers" in order to demonstrate their desire to be identified with education, research, and advancing technology. Within a few years, university medical centers began to call attention to their even higher status by using the name "health sciences center" to distinguish a cluster of professional schools that shared basic science teaching resources and a teaching hospital with these ubiquitous medical centers.

The AMA and Local Coalitions for Medical Education

The leaders of the AMA gradually adjusted to the growing political strength of academic doctors and their allies. In 1956, for example, the AMA Council on Medical Service, adjudicating a complaint, asserted that academic doctors who received salaries and a proportion of the fees charged on their behalf did not compete unfairly with community doctors. But the AMA would not abandon its fervent belief in doctors' autonomy. Thus the council concluded, hollowly, that it did not condone the corporate practice of medicine.[9]

---

[8] Surgeon General's Consulting Group, *Physicians, passim.*

[9] Edward L. Turner, W. S. Wiggins, G. R. Shepherd, "Medical Education in the United States and Canada," 56th Annual Report, *Journal of the American Medical Association*, October 9, 1956, 161: 1651-1653.

191

AMA leaders also stopped insisting that there was no shortage of doctors. In 1951, the House of Delegates had condemned estimates by federal officials that additional physicians were needed.[10] The AMA's chief economist reported that, because output per physician had increased at least one-third between 1940 and 1950, there was a potential oversupply of physicians.[11] In 1954, however, the AMA Council on Medical Education and Hospitals insisted that demand for doctors and other medical personnel was increasing and that new medical schools should, therefore, be established.[12] In 1958, the AMA decided to support legislation for federal grants to medical schools to construct educational facilities. In 1961, it established a loan fund of $12.5 million for medical students. That year, an AMA economist, embarrassed to discover that his predecessor's prediction of an imminent surplus of doctors was still valid, explained that the idea of equality of opportunity justified AMA support for medical school expansion.[13]

The AMA decided there was a shortage of doctors at a time when considerable data suggested that there was no basis for predicting an impending shortage.[14] Between 1950 and 1960, the number of doctors had increased at about the same rate as the population.[15] There was evidence that shortages were limited to particular specialties or geographic regions.[16] Studies of doctors' productivity in both Britain and the United States found that the standard meas-

[10] "Policy of the American Medical Association Regarding the Production of Physicians," *ibid.*, June 30, 1951, 146: 865.

[11] Frank G. Dickinson, "Supply of Physicians' Services," *ibid.*, April 21, 1951, 145: 1264.

[12] U.S. Congress, House, Committee on Interstate and Foreign Commerce, Staff Report, *Medical School Inquiry*, 85th Congress, 1st Session (Washington, D.C.: USGPO, September 1957), 35, quoting the AMA Council on Medical Education and Hospitals: "there will be a constant and continuous demand for increased numbers of medical personnel . . . this will necessitate new medical schools."

[13] Jacob P. Meerman, "Some Comments on the Predicted Future Shortage of Physicians," *Journal of the American Medical Association*, September 16, 1961, 177: 799.

[14] The most frequently quoted estimates of future shortages were those prepared by the Public Health Service according to standards based on the Lee-Jones equation: Joseph W. Mountin, Elliott H. Pennell, Anne G. Berger, *Health Services Areas: Estimates of Future Physician Requirements* Public Health Service Bulletin no. 305 (Washington, D.C.: USGPO, 1949). The estimates were updated in William H. Stewart and Maryland Y. Pennel, "Health Manpower, 1930-75," *Public Health Reports*, March 1960, 75: 174-280.

[15] Margaret D. West, "Manpower for the Health Field: What Are the Prospects?" *Hospitals*, September 16, 1963, 37: 82-88.

[16] Isidore Altman, "Changes in Physician-Population Ratios among the States," *Public Health Reports*, December 1961, 76: 1051-1055.

ures of shortage, doctor-to-population ratios, were crude and misleading indicators.[17]

Many doctors wanted to believe that there was a shortage. Predictions of a shortage helped to persuade state legislators to finance medical education. Moreover, if there were more doctors competing for patients, more of them might practice in small towns and rural areas. In addition, some leaders of organized medicine seem to have believed that, because more doctors would make medical care more accessible, there would be less clamor for national health insurance.

Many doctors linked their conviction that a shortage existed to their fear that medicine was declining in status. Expanding the profession, some argued, would increase its prestige. A Minnesota doctor who had helped to link academic and community colleagues during the 1950s and who advocated federal subsidy of medical schools, argued in an influential book that the profession was not as important as it had been in 1930 or 1940.[18] Doctors frequently told each other at meetings that they were losing prestige. Many doctors asserted, for example, that they were criticized unfairly in the press and on television. Many doctors were conscious of a new time of hostility toward the profession in the media, which, as one historian remarked, no longer gratefully placed them on pedestals.[19] Other doctors worried that the declining quality of medical students threatened to result in even lower status for the profession in the

[17] Antonio Ciocco, Isidore Altman, T. David Truan, "Patient Load and Volume of Medical Services," *Public Health Reports*, June 1952, 67: 527-531. The earliest studies were Antonio Ciocco and Isidore Altman, "Statistics on the Patient Load of Physicians in Private Practice," *Journal of the American Medical Association*, February 13, 1943, 506-513: and A. Ciocco, Burnet M. Davis, and I. Altman, "Measures of Medical Resources and Requirements," *Medical Care*, November 1943, 3: 314-326. British studies are summarized in J. R. Butler, *How Many Patients: A Study of List Size in General Practice*, Occasional Papers in Social Administration no. 64 (London: Bedford Square Press, 1980). Altman agreed, with caution, that a shortage existed in "On Measuring the Need for Physicians," *Medical Times*, November 1961, 89: 1133-1140. Rashi Fein, "Studies in Physician Supply and Distribution," *American Journal of Public Health*, May 1954, 44: 615-624. Cf. Eli Ginzberg, in National Manpower Council, *A Policy for Scientific and Professional Manpower* (New York: Columbia University Press, 1953). Cf. George W. Bachman, "A Method for Measuring Physician Requirements, with Appraisal of Former Methods," *Journal of the American Medical Association*, June 4, 1955, 148: 375-381.

[18] Richard M. Magraw, *Ferment in Medicine* (Philadelphia: W. B. Saunders, 1966). Cf. British Medical Association, *Recruitment to the Medical Profession* (London: BMA, May 1962), 7.

[19] John C. Burnham, "American Medicine's Golden Age: What Happened to It? *Science*, 19 March 1982, 215: 1475-1476.

future. Some doctors complained that bright students interested in the sciences were accepting fellowships to study for Ph.D. degrees under the National Defense Education Act. Many were distressed because their sons rejected medicine as a career. An Iowa surgeon quoted a colleague's son to a national meeting: "Dad has already given up the fight. I feel I want no part of it."[20]

Lobbyists for hospitals and voluntary associations dedicated to research and treatment for particular diseases welcomed doctors' enthusiasm for expanding medical education. Together with academic doctors and many specialty societies, these groups advocated federal support for medical schools' capital and operating budgets with new vigor in the late 1950s. Their allies in Congress and the National Institutes of Health commissioned reports to document and publicize the cause. Like the members of the Guillebaud committee in Britain a few years earlier, the authors of these reports projected beliefs about the past into the future. For example, in 1957, staff members of the House Committee on Interstate and Foreign Commerce justified federal aid to medical education by summarizing the achievements of medicine since the nineteenth century.[21] A year later, a committee told the secretary of health, education, and welfare that the accomplishments of medical research in the past made it necessary to increase subsidies for research and education in the present.[22] Similar assertions had been made in reports for many years. Now, however, they justified the agenda of a national coalition with roots in state and local affairs. The members of this coalition understood the levers—and the limits—of power in American politics.

ORGANIZED MEDICINE AND THE LABOR MOVEMENT

Organized medicine and the labor movement began to work together in the 1950s. Their mutual accommodation was evident initially in doctors' diminishing antagonism toward prepaid group practice. The involvement of the unions in medical practice was a consequence of the growth of voluntary health insurance. Most

[20] These generalizations are based on a sampling of state medical journals from the late 1950s and early 1960s. The quotations are from an issue of the *Journal of the International College of Surgeons* devoted to "A National Emergency: Ways of Meeting the Physician Shortage," September 1961, 36: 395-414.

[21] U.S. Congress, *Medical School Inquiry*, xiii.

[22] The Secretary's Consultants on Medical Research and Education, *The Advancement of Medical Research and Education Through the Department of Health, Education and Welfare* (Washington, D.C.: Office of the Secretary, DHEW, June 27, 1958), 19.

health insurance was purchased by employers from Blue Cross/ Blue Shield or commercial companies, either as a result of collective bargaining or as a way to deter unionization. By 1959, 4 percent of the total compensation of working Americans was paid by employers for health programs.[23] Which services were paid for by health insurance was a matter of enormous importance to hospitals and doctors as well as to labor leaders and workers. Hospital trustees and administrators were eager to increase the costs they could recover, doctors wanted high and stable incomes, and union officials wanted to satisfy their members. Business executives were also concerned about the services covered by health insurance, but mainly as members of hospital and Blue Cross boards.[24]

Union officials became increasingly critical of the behavior of doctors and hospitals during the 1950s. In 1953, for example, an official of the United Automobile Workers complained that, because Blue Cross did not control the costs hospitals passed on to consumers, it put economic pressure on its subscribers.[25] Labor leaders disliked, as an economist wrote in 1959, negotiating benefits that raised the income of doctors and hospitals without expanding the services provided to their members. Several unions organized clinics that were staffed by salaried doctors as alternatives to fee-for-service medicine: the seamen, machinists, and the automobile, ladies garment, amalgamated clothing and mine workers, for instance. In California, Oregon, and the state of Washington, union members constituted the majority of members of prepaid health plans which owned their own hospitals. Municipal workers' unions helped to create the Health Insurance Plan of Greater New York.[26]

[23] Walter Galenson and Robert S. Smith, "The United States," in John T. Dunlop and Walter Galenson, eds., *Labor in the Twentieth Century* (New York: Academic Press, 1978), 59. *Cf.* Duncan M. MacIntyre, *Voluntary Health Insurance and Rate Making* (Ithaca, New York: Cornell University Press, 1962), 11.

[24] No single source examines the history of fringe benefits for medical care as a deliberate public policy choice in the United States. The most comprehensive study is Raymond Munts, *Bargaining for Health: Labor Unions, Health Insurance and Medical Care* (Madison: University of Wisconsin Press, 1967). Paul Starr, *The Social Transformation of American Medicine* (New York: Basic Books, 1982), 315-334, is a useful summary of this history. MacIntyre provides useful historical data in the context of a study of alternative methods of rate making. J. F. Follman, *Medical Care and Health Insurance* (Homewood, Ill.: Richard D. Irwin, 1963), is a useful survey with a bias toward the insurance industry. *Cf.* A. Norman Somers and Louis Schwartz, "Pension and Welfare Plans: Gratuities or Compensation," *Industrial and Labor Relations Review*, October 1952, 4: 77-88.

[25] Munts, *Bargaining for Health*, 72.

[26] Joseph W. Garbarino, *Health Plans and Collective Bargaining* (Berkeley: University

Staff members of unions and of medical associations began to work together to solve practical problems. One union official remarked sympathetically that the semantic problems of the AMA were similar to those of any organization whose members had diverse and conflicting interests.[27] In turn, the general manager of the AMA, explained that union-sponsored prepaid health plans should be permitted to try to do a better job than fee-for-service practice in particular situations.[28] In 1951, the AMA invited doctors employed by unions to join a new Committee on Medical Care for Industrial Workers. In 1953, this committee set "Standards of Acceptance for Medical Care Plans"; two years later, it established "Principles for Evaluation and Management of Union Health Centers." Although many county medical societies in the Appalachian region refused to grant membership—and therefore denied hospital privileges—to doctors employed by the United Mine Workers, the *Journal* of the AMA hoped that organized medicine and union leaders would learn to work amicably together.[29]

The AMA and its affiliates adjusted to the diversity of medical practice. The members of a few state and county medical societies agreed to tolerate prepaid group practice as a result of pressure from doctors who depended for their livelihoods on union benefit plans. In Michigan, for instance, the Wayne County Medical Society was embarrassed when the state society attacked the health plan sponsored by the Automobile Workers. Members of the medical society in San Joaquin, California, organized a foundation to manage a prepayment plan in response, they said, to growing union interest in closed panels.[30] When the members of the medical society in Brooklyn, New York, decided to discriminate against doctors who were employed by the Health Insurance Plan of Greater New York, the AMA Judicial Council advised them to desist because they were violating federal antitrust laws. In 1957, the president of the AMA was, for the first time, an employee of a prepaid group practice. Two years later, an AMA commission urged doctors

---

of California Press, 1960), 35. Munts, *Bargaining for Health*, 150ff.; MacIntyre, *Voluntary Health Insurance, passim*.

[27] Munts, *Bargaining for Health*, 161.

[28] F.J.L. Blasingame, in 1958, quoted in Richard Carter, *The Doctor Business* (Garden City, N.Y.: Doubleday and Co., 1958), 155.

[29] Munts, *Bargaining for Health*, 160, 254. On the influence of collective bargaining on debates about health policy, [Jerome Pollack] "A Labour View of Health Insurance," *Monthly Labor Review*, June 1958, 81: 626-630.

[30] Munts, *Bargaining for Health*, 76, 154.

to regard with tolerance innovations in the organization of medical services. Most important, in 1959 the House of Delegates redefined the principle that patients be permitted a free choice of physician to include their right to choose a group practice.[31]

By 1960, symbolism and service had become conflicting goals within organized medicine. This conflict was evident even though the AMA continued to issue propaganda and many doctors discriminated against colleagues employed by group practices financed by prepayment. For thirty years, the politics of symbolism had united most doctors, who wanted to be accountable only to individual patients and nearby colleagues. The politics of service had supported the politics of symbolism for most of that time. In return for paying dues to their medical society and performing a few political chores, doctors had been guaranteed that government officials would deal with them infrequently and favorably.

During and after World War II, however, doctors increasingly wanted action from government. They wanted specialty training subsidized under the G.I. Bill of Rights, generous reimbursement with which new and enlarged hospitals could hire more staff and purchase equipment, and new and expanded medical schools. Medical societies now served their members by lobbying for subsidies and negotiating for regulations so that doctors could maintain or increase their control of medical care and their share of its price. Symbolic politics can be, sometimes must be, conducted alone; the politics of public subsidy requires allies.

A NATIONAL COALITION

The goals of advocates of national health policy who identified themselves as liberals—mainly union officials, leaders of voluntary health groups, a few academics, and some state and federal civil servants—changed during the 1950s. To some extent this change was a result of the failure to enact national health insurance. But it was also in part a response to the growing strength of local coali-

---

[31] *Ibid.*, 159, 163; Odin W. Anderson, *The Uneasy Equilibrium: Private and Public Financing of Health Services in the United States, 1878-1965* (New Haven: College and University Press, 1968), 161. The antagonism of organized medicine to prepaid group practice declined but it hardly disappeared. Until the late 1970s, doctors who practiced in what were renamed health maintenance organizations were often ostracized by the medical community and accused of unethical behavior. Organized medicine was also able to influence federal and state legislation governing HMOs, making it more difficult for them to operate.

197

tions demanding state and federal subsidy for hospitals and medical education. The liberal lobbies shared much of the agenda of these local coalitions. More important, union leaders, officials of voluntary associations and many experts on medical care abandoned the campaign for national health insurance in order to support medical care for the elderly under Social Security. To some of its advocates, what would be called Medicare was an expedient, a first step toward a comprehensive program. However, many proponents of medical care for the elderly did not regard it as a temporary measure. The elderly, they declared, were unique because, although they needed more medical care than any other group, they could not negotiate for medical benefits through collective bargaining.[32]

The national policy agendas of other pressure groups had also changed by 1960. Officials of the American Hospital Association frequently supported public subsidies to reduce its members' deficits, even though they antagonized the leaders of organized medicine. In the late 1950s, the AHA, led by George Bugbee, began to promote area-wide health planning as a way to focus the attention of local coalitions on the need for state and national policies to reduce hospitals' deficits and promote hierarchical regionalism. Again Bugbee collaborated with officials of the Public Health Service, as he had done to promote the Hill-Burton Act a decade and a half earlier.[33] Moreover, many doctors regretted the AMA's position on national health policy. The Association of American Medical Colleges and specialty societies spoke for an increasing number of doctors, many of whom had acquired political influence. In addition, third-party payers—Blue Cross, Blue Shield, and insurance companies—were eager to have their most expensive risks, elderly and disabled patients, subsidized by public funds.

Prominent social scientists analyzed and applauded the coalition

[32] A participant in these events, Wilbur J. Cohen, emphasized the roots of social policy during the 1960s in the previous decade, in Robert H. Haveman, ed., *A Decade of Federal Antipoverty Programs* (New York: Academic Press, 1977), 189. *Cf.* Martha Derthick, *Policymaking for Social Security* (Washington, D.C.: Brookings Institution, 1979), *passim*.

[33] Commission on Financing Hospital Care, *Financing Hospital Care in the United States*, vol. 3: *Financing Hospital Care for Nonwage and Low Income Groups* (New York: Blakiston-McGraw Hill, 1955). Joint Committee of the American Hospital Association and the Public Health Service, *Areawide Planning for Hospitals and Related Facilities*, PHS Publication no. 855 (Washington, D.C.: USGPO, July 1961); *cf.* Report of the National Commission on Community Health Services, *Health Is a Community Affair* (Cambridge: Harvard University Press, 1966).

supporting federal legislation to increase the supply of health services and to subsidize some of the demand for them. V. O. Key, a leading scholar of pressure-group politics, for example, was confident that subsidized health insurance would be enacted and that doctors could dominate how it was administered.[34] Talcott Parsons, an eminent sociologist, assured the AMA in 1958 that public and private interests were increasingly in harmony. Private health insurance would, he insisted, inevitably grow and would hasten the integration of medicine with society.[35]

A study by Herman and Anne Somers, *Doctors, Patients and Health Insurance*, published in 1961 by the Brookings Institution, was a manifesto for a new coalition. This coalition would unite supporters of hierarchical regionalism with advocates of entitlement programs to pay for care for some individuals. Doctors, they argued, were gaining power to sustain life at a rapidly accelerating rate. The benefits of this power could be extended to more people as a result of public investment in manpower, facilities, and research, public subsidy to provide care for the poor and the elderly, and more extensive voluntary insurance for workers and their dependents. The coalition pressing these policies, the Somers said, should take advantage of the fragmentation of the medical profession and ignore doctrinaire advocates of national health insurance.[36]

The program described by the Somers was widely supported by the press and on television. The media insisted that a crisis existed in medical care and that the remedy for it was regulated growth and targeted subsidy in order to manage in the public interest what a CBS-TV special on "The Business of Health" in 1961 called an "explosion" of technical and scientific progress.[37]

[34] V. O. Key, Jr. *Politics, Parties and Pressure Groups* (New York: Thomas Y. Crowell Co., 1942, 1969), 125-126.

[35] Talcott Parson, "Some Trends of Change in American Society: Their Bearing on Medical Education," *Journal of the American Medical Association*, May 3, 1958, 167: 31-36.

[36] Herman M. Somers and Anne R. Somers, *Doctors, Patients and Health Insurance* (Washington, D.C.: Brookings Institution, 1961), xi, 532, 460, and *passim*. The Somers documented the work of the coalition whose cause they advocated; noting, for example, that the AMA sought to negotiate with organized labor over national policy (243) and quoting Osler Peterson's view that "some of the public opponents of governmental health insurance for the aged, in fact, privately supported it" (449).

[37] CBS Reports, "The Business of Health: Medicine, Money and Politics," February 2, 1961. Script in Michael M. Davis Papers, C-1, New York Academy of Medicine. The combination of awe about medical progress and concern over its increasing cost permeated public discourse in the late 1950s. Thus, in a report to Congress, Morkley Roberts declared that "medical care is becoming wonderfully effective and appal-

President John F. Kennedy responded to the growing cohesion of a coalition advocating new federal policy for medical care. In February 1961, his administration proposed legislation to build hospitals and community mental health centers, increase the number of health professionals, and provide medical care for the elderly under Social Security. This program stalled in Congress, however, and was not a priority of the administration until after the congressional elections of 1962.

The campaign, which accelerated in 1963, to enact what became the Health Professions Educational Assistance Act, demonstrated the strength of the coalition advocating new health policy. In his 1963 State of the Union Address, President Kennedy warned that what he called the "miracles of medical research" would not be disseminated if the growing shortage of doctors and other health professionals was not reversed.[38] The assertion that there was a manpower shortage was unchallenged during extensive congressional hearings over two years. Federal subsidies for construction at professional schools and for aid to students were endorsed by medical, dental, hospital, public health, and group practice associations, farm and labor organizations, and voluntary associations concerned with particular diseases. The Student American Medical Association, disagreeing with its parent organization, joined in advocating federal financial aid to students.

When the bill to subsidize the education of health professionals stalled in Congress, the secretary of health, education, and welfare insisted that it was an essential element of a comprehensive program to increase the supply of medical services. More money for health manpower, Secretary Celebrezze told the Senate Committee on Labor and Public Welfare, was a prerequisite to future advances in all fields of health.[39] These advances would be paid for, he said, by economic growth rather than by redistributing resources. The senators and other witnesses agreed with the Administration that

---

lingly expensive"; Trends in the Supply and Demand of Medical Care," Study Paper no. 5, U.S. Congress, Joint Economic Committee, November 10, 1959 (Washington, D.C.: USGPO, 1959). *Cf.* "The Crisis in American Medicine," A Special Supplement of *Harper's*, October, 1960, 221: 123-168; *cf.* Burnham, "Medicine's Golden Age."

[38] State of the Union Address, *Congressional Record*, House of Representatives, 88th Congress, 1st Session, vol. 109, Part I, January 14, 1963, 172.

[39] U.S. Congress, House, Committee on Interstate and Foreign Commerce, 88th Congress, 1st session, *Health Professions Educational Assistance*, H.R. 12, etc., February 5, 6, 7, 1963, 37.

an expanding national economy and additional personal savings as a result of better health would pay the cost of new policy.[40]

IMPLEMENTING CONSENSUS

Between 1964 and 1966, Lyndon Johnson and the 89th Congress wrote into law the policies advocated by the coalition that had grown since World War II. The rapid enactment of so much new legislation was the result of events outside health politics. When John Kennedy was assassinated, in November 1963, the Health Professions Educational Assistance Act and a program to create community mental health centers were the only practical achievements of the health program of his Administration. Lyndon Johnson's political skills, his popularity, and the election of an unusual number of liberal congressmen in the Democratic landslide of November 1964 persuaded the chairmen of powerful committees in the House and Senate that there was enormous support for the Administration's domestic program, and for its health legislation in particular.[41]

The extraordinary political situation between 1963 and 1966 explains the rapid enactment but not the substance of the Johnson Administration's health program. In the United States in 1965, as in Britain in 1946, events in general politics and society made it possible for widely shared beliefs about the value and the organization of medical care to become, for a time, more important than considerations of party and group interest. Although lobbyists, Administration officials, and the members and staff of congressional committees negotiated at length about the details of each of the new health programs, they agreed about their purpose. As in Britain in 1946, policy to remove barriers, especially financial impediments, to access was combined with policy to improve the quality of care by increasing and reorganizing the supply of services. The Great Society,

[40] *Ibid.* 54, for Chairman Oren Harris stating that growth rather than taxes would finance health policy. U.S. Congress, Senate . . . Hearings on S.911 and H.R. 12, *Medical, Dental and Public Health Teaching Facilities,* August 22, 23, 26, 1963 (Washington, D.C.: USGPO, 1963), 62.

[41] The liberalism of the 89th Congress was, however, mainly the result of a gradual change in its membership rather than of the Johnson landslide. Like the coalition for a national health program, the coalition of liberals in Congress had developed gradually, particularly as a result of the numerical growth in liberal senators after 1958; Michael Foley, *The New Senate: Liberal Influence on a Conservative Institution, 1959-1972* (New Haven: Yale University Press, 1980).

like the postwar Labour Government, though in different ways, linked equity with hierarchical regionalization.

During the Johnson Administration, shared beliefs and the practical experience of coalition in the recent past made possible unprecedented alliances in support of new health policy. The new politics of health affairs was evident during hearings on the Hill-Burton program in the closing days of the 88th Congress in 1964. Most interest groups, including the American Hospital Association and the AMA, agreed that federal hospital policy should now give priority in funding to cities and in particular to teaching hospitals. Congressmen and their witnesses discussed hospital construction in the context of proposals, which they assumed would be enacted, to remedy shortages of manpower and to subsidize hospital care for the aged and indigent.[42] In the workshops of American politics, though not yet in the press, on television, or in the forums in which the AMA's staff consoled the remnants of its grass roots constituency, the United States was moving toward a new national health policy.

Lyndon Johnson's message to Congress announcing his health program proclaimed familiar goals. The health of the people, the president said, should be the foundation for fulfilling Americans' aspirations. His policy was the result, he continued, of a great and continuing revolution in medical knowledge. The potential for health in the future was unlimited, he concluded, because science was now linked to achieving equity; to a national commitment that the advance of medical knowledge should leave none behind.[43]

Similar goals had been proclaimed for a generation by presidents, leaders of interest groups, and the media. For some participants in health politics, these words were articles of faith; for others, they were self-evident platitudes that justified aggrandizing the interests they represented. For the first time, however, the assumption that properly organized and distributed medical care linked to entitlement programs which paid for services for the elderly and the poor

[42] U.S. Congress, House, Committee on Interstate and Foreign Commerce, *Extension and Revision of Hill-Burton Hospital Construction Program*, 88th Congress, 2nd Session, Hearing, March 1964 (Washington, D.C.: USGPO, May 1964), 46, 122, 127, 135, 182, 227, 252-255. No objections were recorded when Surgeon General Luther Terry admitted (155) that the government based its policy on self-surveys by the hospital industry: each institution determined its own "need" for alteration, renovation, and new construction.

[43] "Advancing the Nation's Health-Message from the President of the United States," *Congressional Record*, 89th Congress, 1st session, vol. III, Part I, January 7, 1965, 407, 408, 411.

would lead to social progress was embodied in a program that was supported by an effective national coalition.[44]

The president spoke for a coalition that was rooted in state and local affairs and had twenty years of political experience. The members of the coalition agreed on the substance of a program to subsidize the supply of medical services and, to a more limited extent, the demand for them. Only the elderly would be entitled to receive medical care subsidized with public funds without undergoing a means test. As a result of the series of accommodations which, in 1965, were enacted as Medicaid, the states would continue to determine which of their residents who were not privately insured or who had exhausted Medicare benefits would receive what medical services. For everyone except the elderly covered by Medicare, therefore, it became national policy that access to services would vary widely as a result of decisions by the states about the poor and by private insurers about everyone else. The federal government would offer incentives to the states to offer particular benefits and would mandate a minimum level of services for the people whom the states chose to make eligible for Medicaid.

A commitment to hierarchical regionalism was so fundamental to the coalition that it was rarely articulated. Almost everyone seemed to assume that subsidies for the supply of services—for research, professional education, hospital construction, and comprehensive health planning—would reinforce and make more efficient the organization of services in appropriate hierarchical levels in each medical care region. Similarly, subsidies for demand—Medicare and Medicaid—would be spent by elderly and poor consumers at proper levels within regional hierarchies as a result of rational planning for access to care and systematic review of hospital utilization by peer groups and planning agencies.

Only the American Medical Association was outside the coalition, and then only about Medicare.[45] The AMA made Medicare a

---

[44] The most accessible accounts of the medical care legislation of the 1960s are in Congressional Quarterly Service, *Congress and the Nation*, vols. I and II (Washington, D.C.: Congressional Quarterly Service, 1965, 1969): vol. I, 1113-1158; vol. II, 665-704. *Cf.* Herman M. and Anne R. Somers, *Medicare and the Hospitals* (Washington, D.C.: Brookings Institution, 1967), *passim*. *Cf.* Rufus E. Miles, Jr., *Awakening From the American Dream* (New York: Universe Books, 1976). *Cf.* Starr, *Social Transformation*, 363-378.

[45] The AMA endorsed each new program except Medicare. For example: U.S. Congress, House, Committee on Interstate and Foreign Commerce, 89th Congress, 2nd session, *Comprehensive Planning and Public Health Services: Amendments of 1966*, October 11, 1966 (Washington, D.C.: USGPO, December 1966), 58-68. Bargaining within

symbol for a definition of autonomy that had become an anachronism to many doctors.[46] During the controversy over Medicare, AMA leaders frequently said that doctors' offices rather than hospitals should be the focus of medical care in the United States.[47] In order to preserve doctors' right to practice in isolation, AMA leaders committed fundamental errors of political tactics—for instance, campaigning against Senator Lister Hill in Alabama in 1962 and irritating Wilbur Mills, chairman of the House Ways and Means Committee, in 1965 by preaching to him about doctors' autonomy during hearings on technical issues.[48] As had happened in Britain in 1947, some medical leaders threatened a boycott of Medicare, even though most doctors said that they would accept patients under the new program.

Once Medicare was enacted, the AMA quickly rejoined the national coalition advocating health policy. James Appel, the AMA president-elect, told his colleagues that they must be active in negotiations over regulations to implement Medicare in order to represent the divergent points of view among members of the profession.[49] Edward Annis, who had been the AMA's most prominent spokesman against Medicare, put it more crudely; doctors must, he

---

the consensus and the achievement of near unanimity on each measure has been documented with particular clarity for the Regional Medical Program: Elinor Langer, "Presidential Medicine," *Science*, March 20, 1964, 142: 1308-1309; John M. Russell, "New Federal Regional Medical Programs," *New England Journal of Medicine*, August 11, 1965, 275: 309-312; *cf.* David E. Price, *Who Makes the Laws? Creativity and Power in Senate Committees* (Cambridge: Schenkman Publishing Co., 1972), 220ff.

[46] Urologists, for instance, in a national meeting, repeated violent rhetoric of AMA denunciations of Medicare (including what may, perhaps, be their unique concern that "the medical profession faces emasculation"), and concluded that the Blue Shield Professional Service Index for calculating fees by specialty "will [and should be] a factor in all future legislation pertinent to medical care, whether it be voluntary or involuntary." (Donald Jaffer *et al.*, "Socio-Economic Problems Confronting the Members of the American Urological Association," *Journal of Urology*, April 1963, 89: 628-637.)

[47] Max J. Skidmore, *Medicare and the American Rhetoric of Reconciliation* (Montgomery: University of Alabama Press, 1970), 140.

[48] On Hill, Price, *Who Makes the Laws?* 223-224; on Mills, Theodore R. Marmor, *The Politics of Medicare* (Chicago: Aldine, 1970), 66.

[49] James Z. Appel, "We the People of the U.S.—Are We Sheep?" *Journal of the American Medical Association*, July 5, 1965, 193: 26-30. Two months later, medical involvement in expanding Medicare to cover doctors' fees was documented by Arlen J. Large, "How Doctors Helped Expand Medicare," *Medical Economics*, September 6, 1965, 42: 259-289. On the accommodation of American doctors to whatever residual discomfort they had to Medicare, see Judith M. Feder, *Medicare: The Politics of Federal Hospital Insurance* (Lexington, Mass.: D.C. Health and Co., 1977), *passim*.

insisted, get inside the enemy camp.[50] The Johnson administration welcomed the AMA into the national coalition, amending a bill to create regional medical programs—a measure to diffuse knowledge through hierarchies eminating from medical schools and teaching hospitals—in order to please the association just a few months after Dr. Appel's speech.[51]

In the summer of 1965, a consensus about health policy was supported by a larger and more powerful coalition in the United States than at any time in the past. Commenting on what had been achieved by this coalition, the surgeon general of the Public Health Service, William Stewart, said that its success revealed that diversity was the great strength of American society. Because of diversity, no single element of the coalition, neither private nor academic medicine nor government could, he said, "write a prescription for policy and impose it" on other groups.[52]

For the moment, diversity was coordinated and harmonized by what Dr. Stewart described as a partnership. Industry, labor, many doctors, hospital associations, Blue Cross and the insurance industry, and eventually organized medicine had coalesced to support the president's program. For the first time, a president had put relentless pressure on members of Congress to enact a program to increase and rationalize the supply of medical care and to subsidize demand for it by the elderly and the poor. In Congress, the president's—that is, the coalition's—program was supported by both optimistic liberals and chastened conservatives. Many of the elderly and some of the poor had joined new political organizations whose leaders pressed their claims alongside allies in the health professions, government, and the industrial and labor lobbies.

Dr. Stewart and most of his contemporaries believed that the consensus about health policy was the result of more than shared self-interest among allies in the coalition. Health, in Stewart's metaphor, was interwoven into the fabric of American culture. Nevertheless, the health partnership could not, he warned, impose policy without restraint. The people themselves, through their values, Stewart said, would determine the ultimate design of health policy.[53]

[50] Skidmore, *Medicare*, 141.

[51] Richard A. Rettig, *Cancer Crusade* (Princeton: Princeton University Press, 1977), 39.

[52] William H. Stewart, "Education for the Health Professions," White House Conference on Health, November 3, 1965, quoted in John M. Knowles, ed., *The Teaching Hospital* (Cambridge: Harvard University Press, 1966), 5.

[53] *Ibid.*, 5.

The leaders of the coalition that had created a national health program did not speculate in 1965, at least not in public, about whether the value Americans assigned to achieving health by investing in more medical care was likely to change. For the moment, members of the health professions, leaders of the hospital industry, third-party payers, business executives, labor union officials, and the most prominent politicians in the nation were united by shared beliefs and mutual self-interest. This coalition had emerged gradually, often tortuously, during the previous half-century and then, with a great rush, translated its agenda into national policy.

In the mid-1960s, health policy seemed to many people in Britain and the United States to be a logical result of the progress of medicine. Because of health policy, it seemed, medical research and practice had reduced deaths and relieved suffering from many diseases. Because medical care was distributed through hierarchies of institutions and professionals in geographic regions, it would, according to this vision, conquer more diseases in the future. Moreover, the aspirations of working- and middle-class people for greater equity in the distribution of wealth and a higher standard of living had become social policy in each nation. In both nations, some people criticized the cost, the effectiveness, and the equity of health policy. Most of the critics believed, however, that these problems would be solved when more resources were appropriated and services were organized more efficiently. Most people, satisfied with the results of the history of health policy in the first seven decades of the century, were confident that they knew how to prepare for the future.

The Consequences of
Hierarchical Regionalism

THIS BOOK is a history of ideas about organizing health policy and of the priority accorded to organization in health policy because of those ideas. In the mid-1960s, as a result of the ideas I have described, many people in Britain and the United States were confident that medical science would continue to progress and be disseminated efficiently through regional hierarchies. Since the 1960s, however, health policy based on hierarchical regionalism has had unexpected consequences.

Belief in the continuous progress of medical science and its applications was rooted in the nineteenth century. In the last half of that century, increasing numbers of people became convinced that medical science could provide them with unprecedented benefits. This widely shared belief in the growing effectiveness of medical care stimulated a profound change in health policy in Britain and the United States. In both countries, the goal of policy to improve citizens' health became the increase of access to medical procedures. Higher priority was accorded to finding disease and alleviating its effects than to creating more healthful environments or to better nutrition or to providing money to replace wages lost through illness.

In both countries, moreover, a consensus grew that medical services should be organized in regional hierarchies. This hierarchy was justified by the process by which the unprecedented progress of medical science had occurred. New discoveries were made in the laboratories of research institutes and medical schools and were applied initially to patients in the wards of teaching hospitals. This knowledge was then disseminated to settings of gradually decreasing technical sophistication: to general and special hospitals, clinics and health centers, doctors' offices and patients' homes. The goal of policy became the subsidization of planning, construction, and management of linked institutions, particularly of hospitals, in particular geographic regions.

These institutional hierarchies were logical expressions of the way tasks were organized within the medical profession for most of

207

the twentieth century. Some doctors created knowledge; others specialized in applying sophisticated techniques; most of them mediated between their colleagues and members of the public and treated complaints that did not require specialized attention. Medical knowledge apparently flowed down hierarchies serving particular geographic regions; patients should, in theory, be referred up the same hierarchies. Knowledge and the ability to command institutional resources became the basis of doctors' standing among their colleagues and patients.

Health policy in both countries was based increasingly on the assumption that medical care would be distributed more equitably and efficiently by regional hierarchies. There were, however, significant differences between American and British motives for reorganizing medical services. Americans frequently acted as if scientific progress, coupled with economic growth, would promote equity. The British emphasized the role of efficient administration, which could be independent of science, in the equitable distribution of resources. Moreover, health policy was compartmentalized in American politics, in part as the price of building effective political coalitions. The British, in contrast, conceived of health care as an element of an integrated social policy that also provided adequate income, decent housing, and accessible social services. Despite these differences, most people in each country have assumed throughout this century that mortality and morbidity rates for populations would decline if more properly organized medical services were provided more frequently for more patients.

This agreement on ends—the widespread belief that more medical care for individuals distributed through regional hierarchies would lead to better health for populations—was obscured by conflict over means in both nations. Debates about how to pay doctors, govern hospitals, and apportion the costs of caring for working-class and indigent patients seemed more important to contemporaries throughout the century than did the consensus about hierarchical regionalism. Almost every participant in these debates agreed, however, that policy should assist progress by allocating more resources to health care.

Similar beliefs led to similar events in Britain and the United States. In each country, governments acted to subsidize research and professional education, increase the supply of professionals and facilities, establish and encourage regional hierarchies, and reduce the direct cost of care to patients. In each, moreover, the press and later radio, movies and television reinforced the consensus that it was in the public interest to allocate more resources to health care.

Health policy was, however, also shaped by the political culture, class relationships, and economic resources of each country. In each, new health policy was advocated and implemented by coalitions whose members belonged to opposing parties, held conflicting political philosophies and had different professional and economic interests. The members of the coalition that created the National Health Service during and after World War II were united by their commitment to the cluster of policies that are usually called the Welfare State. This commitment was reinforced by the doctrines and actions of the major political parties. Moreover, the substance of policy and the timing of its initiation was influenced by the painful experience of two world wars and by the economic and social problems of recovering from them.

In the United States, in contrast, a coalition that was broad enough to create national legislation could only be organized to support a narrower range of policy. The American polity is more fragmented than the British by geography, by economic interests, and by competing beliefs about the role of government in social policy. Most of the groups whose members argued about proper health policy between 1914 and 1940 resisted compromise, even when it could have easily been achieved. During and after World War II, however, a coalition was organized whose adherents promoted subsidies to increase the supply of medical services—beginning with hospitals—and to organize them in loose, often informal, regional hierarchies. This coalition relied on tax policy and economic growth to stimulate effective demand for care. By the 1960s the leaders of this coalition—or, more accurately, of coalitions in states and cities that supported particular national policies—were eager to have the federal government pay the direct cost of care for the elderly and the poor, subsidize increases in the supply of professionals, facilities, and scientific knowledge, and promote state and regional health planning.

Doctors were significant actors, though in different ways, in health policy in both nations. Their decisions determined the allocation of the resources each nation was willing to provide for health services. In Britain, beginning in 1950, an overall ceiling on expenditures for the NHS was set by the government. In the United States, in contrast, the rising costs of medical decisions were passed on to government, insurers, and individual consumers until very recently. American doctors and hospitals enjoyed enormous increases in income in exchange for accommodating to what became, incrementally, a national medical care program. British doctors have also benefited from health policy, but their personal gains were, to a large extent, independent of their decisions about how much care to provide to whom, when, and where.

Hierarchical regionalism remains fundamental to health policy in Britain and the United States. The assumption that knowledge that will lead to better health is usually discovered in university and hospital laboratories continues to guide investment in facilities, equipment, and personnel for medical research and education. The assumption that the results of medical research are disseminated most efficiently down hierarchies dominated by teaching hospitals is still the basis of policy to plan and build general hospitals and health centers and to link doctors to them. The assumption that consumers are entitled to receive services of increasing sophistication and cost continues to drive policy to finance medical care.[1]

However, the success of hierarchical regionalism stimulated the erosion of regional hierarchies beginning in the 1970s. The events of the past two decades are beyond the scope of this book. But a brief, tentative summary of them may be of use to readers who are drawn to history because of their interest in contemporary affairs.

Erosion has occurred more rapidly in the United States than in Britain. Public subsidies for biomedical science, professional education, and improved access to services unintentionally tore apart fragile regional hierarchies. Public sponsorship of biomedical research and its applications caused an unprecedented increase in the number of new drugs, devices, and medical procedures. Subsidies to train more medical specialists increased the number of doctors on the staffs of small and middle-sized hospitals who were able and eager to perform sophisticated procedures. Third-party payers, moreover, reimbursed doctors without regard to their sophistication and hospitals so long as they were accredited. Public programs to plan health systems and subsidize the construction of new facilities were administered by state officials who assumed that efficient regionalization would continue to result from mutual accommodation among institutions, each of which would benefit from the growing resources of the health sector. Public subsidy of the care of elderly and poor patients and tax subsidies for voluntary insurance made

[1] Recent evidence of continuing commitment to hierarchical regionalism is in Jean de Kervasdoue, John R. Kimberly, and Victor G. Rodwin, eds., *The Future of Health Policy in Western Industrialized Nations* (Berkeley: University of California Press, 1984), 9: "In the future, regional health systems with networks linking hospitals and specialists to general practitioners and support services are likely to predominate."

most of the people in every community sources of potential income to doctors and hospitals.

The most important of the unexpected consequences of health policy has been the increasing financial cost of medical care.[2] Sir William Beveridge's optimistic assumption that the advance of medical science would stabilize the costs of diagnosing and treating illness has proven profoundly wrong. So has the hope that economic growth would absorb the increased cost of medical services. In both countries, more people received more services for more afflictions than ever before at a cost that was steadily increasing.

In both Britain and the United States controlling costs became a central goal of health policy in the 1970s. At first, policymakers in both countries tried to use the strategies of hierarchical regionalism, which had been so effective in the years of growth, to restrain the rate at which costs increased. In the United States these efforts included mandated peer review of the inpatient services doctors ordered for Medicare patients, incentives to create health maintenance organizations, certificate of need programs to inhibit new hospital construction and regulate the diffusion of expensive new technology, and the establishment of new regional planning organizations, the Health Systems Agencies. In Britain, the National Health Service, which had been reorganized in 1974 in order to plan growth more rationally, adapted with great difficulty to an "era of economic pessimism."[3] Yet costs continued to escalate. As a result, in both countries the cost crisis assisted the political ascendancy of ideological opponents of universality, risk-pooling, collective provision, and regulation as fundamental principles of social policy.

The regional hierarchies established in the United States since the 1940s are changing rapidly in the 1980s. Regions have become more self-contained. Not only are fewer patients being referred up hierarchies to teaching hospitals, but fewer are now referred outside their regions to such centers of medical research as New York City.[4] Within regions, moreover, hospitals increasingly compete with each other. Large teaching hospitals compete with smaller ones and with community hospitals for patients whose conditions they would have treated just a few years ago. In some areas, investor-owned firms and multi-hospital non-profit organizations manage

[2] Robert J. Maxwell, *Health and Wealth* (Lexington, Mass.: D. C. Heath, 1981).

[3] Rudolf Klein, *The Politics of the National Health Service* (London: Longman, 1983), Chapter 4.

[4] Health Systems Agency of New York City, *Medical Facilities Plan for the City of New York*, vol. 1, December 1983, 66ff.

or own hospitals at several levels of a hierarchy and refer patients within their system.[5]

Similar challenges to hierarchical regionalism have not yet occurred in Britain because the National Health Service is centrally controlled and financed and because it has strong support among adherents of each political party. However, as the NHS regions become more self-contained the teaching hospitals in London treat fewer patients from elsewhere in Britain.[6] Moreover, the government has recently encouraged doctors to perform, in private hospitals, surgical procedures for which profit margins can be high and NHS waiting lists long.[7]

Rising expenditures for medical care and increasing competition among doctors and hospitals are results of the success of hierarchical regionalism. The assumptions on which health policy was based in the past created the problems and opportunities of the present. These assumptions were derived from an interpretation of history; the belief that hierarchical regionalism, a particular method of organizing scientific research and medical care, would promote progress in the future because it had done so in the past.

In both a practical and a philosophical sense, however, there is no past—no correct description of any earlier time. There is only evidence, which historians must reinterpret continuously. Just as there is no past, there is also no future—no way to predict what will happen. There is only a succession of presents, each with enormous possibilities for thought and action. The study of history is a source of experience, not of justifications for policy.

[5] Reliable accounts include; Irving L. Lewis and Cecil G. Sheps, *The Sick Citadel: The American Academic Medical Center and the Public Interest* (Cambridge: Ballinger, 1983), and Bradford H. Gray, ed., *The New Health Care for Profit* (Washington: National Academy Press, 1983). *Cf.* David A. Gee and Lisa A. Rosenfeld, "The Effect on Academic Health Centers of Tertiary Care in Community Hospitals," *Journal of Medical Education*, July 1984, 59: 547-552.

[6] Jane Smith, "Conflict Without Change: The Case of London's Health Services," *Political Quarterly*, October-December 1981, 52: 426-440.

[7] Rudolf Klein, "The Politics of Ideology vs. the Reality of Politics: The Case of Britain's National Health Service in the 1980s," *Milbank Memorial Fund Quarterly: Health and Society*, Winter 1984, 62: 82-109.

I DESCRIBE the most important sources for this book in the following pages, listing primary and secondary sources by chapters. I supply information about publication and the location of archival material the first time I mention each source.

INTRODUCTION

I summarize and assess the literature on the history of health policy and of the welfare state in each country in three papers: "The National Health Service and the Second World War: The Elaboration of Consensus," in Harold L. Smith, ed., *War and Social Change: British Society in the Second World War* (Manchester: Manchester University Press, 1986); "The Decline of Historicism: The Case of Compulsory Health Insurance in the United States," *Bulletin of the History of Medicine*, Winter 1983: 596-609; and "History and Health Policy: An Autobiographical Note on the Decline of Historicism," *Journal of Social History*, March 1985, 18: 349-364. I am critical, but also appreciative, of this literature. I choose, as a matter of style, to present it only in the notes and in this note on sources. The goal of this book is to build upon, not to replace, what many other scholars have done.

I. HEALTH POLICY AND THE PERCEPTION OF MEDICAL PROGRESS, 1910-1918

There are many important secondary sources for changes in how medicine was perceived in the late nineteenth and early twentieth centuries, but as yet no satisfactory explanation for the surge in demand for care. A useful recent book about Britain is F. B. Smith, *The People's Health* (London: Croom Helm, 1979). Paul Starr, *The Social Transformation of American Medicine* (New York: Basic Books, 1982) is an important synthesis of the literature on medical practice in the United States since the nineteenth century. Important recent contributions to the history of how hospitals were perceived in Britain are John Woodward, *To Do the Sick No Harm* (London: Routledge and Kegan Paul, 1974), and Adrian Forty, "The Modern Hospital in England and France: The Social and Medical Uses of Architecture," in Anthony D. King, ed., *Buildings and Society* (London: Routledge and Kegan Paul, 1980). Standish Meacham, *A Life Apart: The English Working Class, 1890-1914* (London: Thames and Hudson, 1977) is a useful survey of attitudes, including those toward health and medical care. For changing perceptions in the United States in this period, the best secondary sources remain the numerous books and papers by Charles Rosenberg. An important synthesis of historians' current knowledge of the effectiveness of medical care is Barbara Gutmann Rosenkrantz, "Damaged Goods: Dilemma of Responsibility for Risk," *Milbank Memorial Fund Quarterly: Health and Society*, Winter 1979, 57: 1-37. See also, John Harley Warner, "The Therapeutic Perspective: Medical Knowledge, Practice, and Professional Identity in America, 1820-1885" (unpublished dissertation, Harvard University, 1984).

There is a rich literature about the fascination with health in various nations in the nineteenth and early twentieth centuries. For Britain: Bruce Haley, *The Healthy Body and Victorian Culture* (Cambridge: Harvard University Press, 1978); Asa Briggs, "Middlemarch and the Doctors," *Cambridge Journal*, September 1948, 1: 749-762; J. M. Mackintosh, *Trends of Opinion about the Public Health, 1901-1951* (London: Oxford University Press, 1953). The United States: Barbara Sicherman, "The New Mission of the Doctor: Redefining Health and Health Care in the Progressive Era, 1900-1917," in William R. Rogers and David Barnard eds., *Nourishing the Humanistic in Medicine* (Pittsburgh: University of Pittsburgh Press, 1979); essays by Sicherman and John Burnham in Jacques Quen and Eric T. Carlson, eds., *American Psychoanalysis: Origins and Development* (New York: Brunner Mazel, 1978); John Burnham, "Psychiatry, Psychology and the Progressive Movement," *American Quarterly*, 1960, 12: 457-465, and "Psychoanalysis and American Medicine, 1894-1918: Medicine, Science and Culture," *Psychological Issues*, 1967, 5: monograph no. 20; Barbara Gutmann Rosenkrantz, *Public Health and the State: Changing Views in Massachusetts* (Cambridge: Harvard University Press, 1972).

The secondary literature about doctors has grown rapidly. M. Jean Peterson, *The Medical Profession in Mid-Victorian London*, synthesizes numerous recent studies about Britain. Also noteworthy is Noël Parry and Jose Parry, *The Rise of the Medical Profession* (London: Croom Helm, 1976). A useful comparative study is Jeffrey L. Berlant, *Profession and Monopoly: A Study of Medicine in the United States and Great Britain* (Berkeley: University of California Press, 1975). For the United States, a good summary is William G. Rothstein, *American Physicians in the 19th Century: From Sect to Science* (Baltimore: Johns Hopkins University Press, 1972). There are numerous local studies; one of the best is Thomas N. Bonner, *Medicine in Chicago, 1850-1950* (Madison: The State Historical Society of Wisconsin, 1957). An important study is James G. Burrow, *Organized Medicine in the Progressive Era: The Move Toward Monopoly* (Baltimore: Johns Hopkins University Press, 1977).

The literature on hospitals includes: for Britain, Brian Abel-Smith, *The Hospitals, 1800-1948* (London: Heinemann, 1964), and its companion volume, Robert Pinker, *English Hospital Statistics* (London: Heinemann, 1966), and John Woodward, *To Do the Sick No Harm*; for the United States, Charles Rosenberg's "And Heal the Sick: The Hospital and Patient in 19th-Century America," *The Journal of Social History*, 1977, 10: 448-487, and "Inward Vision and Outward Glance: The Shaping of the American Hospital, 1880-1914," *Bulletin of the History of Medicine*, Fall 1979, 53: 346-391. Recent local studies of general importance are Morris J. Vogel, *The Invention of the Modern Hospital* (Chicago: University of Chicago Press, 1980); Rosemary Stevens, "Sweet Charity—State Aid to Hospitals in Pennsylvania, 1870-1910," *Bulletin of the History of Medicine*, Fall, Winter, 1984, 58: 287-314, 474-495; and David Rosner, *A Once Charitable Enterprise* (Cambridge: Cambridge University Press, 1982).

The leading secondary sources on social policy and mandatory health insurance are generally well grounded in archival evidence. I have supplemented these sources by sampling the contemporary periodical and pamphlet literature in both nations. In order better to comprehend British intellectual history in the period, I worked in the William Braithwaite and Passfield (Sidney and Beatrice Webb) papers at the London School of Economics and Political Science and the Fabian Society papers at Nuffield College, Oxford.

Secondary sources on social policy in Britain and the United States in the early twentieth century include: Bentley B. Gilbert, *The Evolution of National Insurance in Great Britain* (London: Michael Joseph, 1966); Geoffrey R. Searle, *The Quest for National Efficiency: A Study in British Politics and Social Thought, 1899-1914* (Oxford: Basil Blackwell, 1971); Ronald Numbers, *Almost Persuaded* (Baltimore: Johns Hopkins University Press, 1978), who cites the leading secondary sources for social policy in the United States; and Daniel M. Fox, *The Discovery of Abundance: Simon N. Patten and the Transformation of Social Theory* (Ithaca: Cornell University Press, 1967).

Gilbert and Numbers are now the standard sources for the politics of compulsory health insurance in each nation. Other notable monographs about Britain are: H. V. Emy, *Liberals, Radicals and So-*

cial Politics, 1892-1914 (Cambridge: Cambridge University Press, 1973); J. R. Hay, *The Origins of the Liberal Welfare Reforms, 1906-1914* (London: Macmillan, 1975); an early and still indispensable study is Gertrude Williams, *The State and the Standard of Living* (London: P. S. King, 1936); a challenge to the standard interpretation, which emphasizes Lloyd George's concern with curative medicine is Frank Honigsbaum, *The Struggle for the Ministry of Health* (London: Ball, 1970); useful political biographies are Kenneth O. Morgan, *The Age of Lloyd George* (London: George Allen and Unwin, 1971); and Kenneth and Jane Morgan, *The Political Career of Christopher, Viscount Addison* (Oxford: Clarendon Press, 1980). Studies of the evolution of compulsory insurance in the United States include: Odin Anderson, "Health Insurance in the United States, 1910-1920," *Journal of the History of Medicine and Allied Sciences*, Autumn 1950, 5: 363-396; and Roy Lubove, *The Struggle for Social Security* (Cambridge: Harvard University Press, 1968). Rosemary Stevens, *American Medicine and the Public Interest* (New Haven: Yale University Press, 1971), is an important study of health policy. There is no satisfactory secondary source on the history of regionalism, either in general or in medical care. I have listed some pertinent studies in the notes.

II. Commitment to Hierarchy and Regionalism:
Britain, 1918-1929

The principal primary sources for the history of regionalism in British health policy are: published public documents in the British Library; parliamentary debates; unpublished documents pertaining to the Dawson Report and Sir George Newman's *Diaries*, in the Library of the Department of Health and Social Services, London; the records of committees of the British Medical Association in the BMA Registry, Tavistock House, London; the collection of pamphlets and correspondence in the Labour Party Archives, London; and the pamphlet and periodical literature available in the British Library and the Libraries of the Wellcome Institute and the London School of Hygiene.

Major secondary sources for the issues discussed in this chapter include: for general social policy, Bentley Gilbert, *British Social Policy, 1914-39* (London: B. T. Batsford, 1970), and Arthur Marwick, *Britain in the Century of Total War* (London: The Bodley Head, 1968); for the Ministry of Health, the works by Honigsbaum listed above; for general politics, Kenneth O. Morgan, *Consensus and Disarray: The Lloyd George Coalition Government, 1918-1922* (Oxford: Clarendon Press, 1979), and Kenneth and Jane Morgan's biography of Addison, Ross McKibbon, *The Evolution of the Labour Party, 1910-1924* (London: Oxford University Press, 1974), and Rodney Lowe, "The Erosion of State Intervention in Britain, 1917-1924," *Economic History Review*, May 1978, 31: 270-286; for the history of health policy, Gordon Forsyth, *Doctors and State Medicine* (London: Pitman Medical, 1973); and for the social history of medicine, Jane Lewis, *The Politics of Motherhood: Child and Maternal Welfare in England, 1900-1939* (London: Croom Helm 1980).

III. The Promise and Threat of Hierarchy:
The United States, 1918-1933

Major primary sources include: professional and general periodical literature; papers pertaining to medical education in the Rockefeller Archives, Tarrytown, New York, and the Abraham Flexner Papers, Library of Congress; published reports of other foundations; the Michael M. Davis Papers, New York Academy of Medicine; and the numerous publications of the Committee on the Costs of Medical Care.

I describe debate and action about health policy in these years and pertinent primary sources, in *Economists and Health Care* and "Abraham Flexner's Unpublished Report: Foundations and Medical Education, 1909-1928," *Bulletin of the History of Medicine*, Winter 1980, 54: 475-496. E. Richard Brown, *Rockefeller Medicine Men* (Berkeley: University of California Press, 1979) interprets the foundation sources differently than I do; Daniel M. Fox, "Ideology vs. Methodology," *Bulletin of the History of Medicine*, Winter 1980, 54: 591-593. A major contribution to the history of medical education is Kenneth M. Ludmerer, *Learning to Heal* (New York: Basic Books, 1985).

Other pertinent secondary sources include: on general intellectual history and on W. F. Ogburn in particular, Richard H. Pells, *Radical Visions and the American Dream* (New York: Harper and Row, 1973); on public health, James H. Cassedy, *Charles V. Chapin and the Public Health Movement* (Cambridge: Harvard University Press, 1962), B. Rosenkrantz, *Public Health and the State*, and Arthur Viseltear, "C. E.-A. Winslow: His Era and His Contributions to Medical Care," in Charles E. Rosenberg, ed., *Healing and History* (New York: Science History Publications, 1979).

IV. Strengthening Consensus: Britain, 1929-1939

Primary sources include: for popular culture, a sample of newspapers and magazines, notably the *Daily Express, Daily Herald, Daily*

Mirror, News Chronical, News of the World, Illustrated London News, and a variety of women's magazines cited in the notes; for national policy, Ministry of Health documents in the Public Record Office; for doctors, papers and pamphlets in the BMA Registry, supplemented by memoirs, notably those of Sir Henry Brackenbury and Alfred Cox cited in the notes; for voluntary hospitals, the British Hospitals Contributory Schemes Association Papers at the London School of Economics and Political Science (which, despite their name, are a collection of British Hospital Association documents); for local authorities, reports of the London County Council and other authorities and the papers of the Society of Medical Officers of Health at the Wellcome Unit, Oxford University; for the Left, publications of the Socialist Medical Association and material in the Labour Party Archives; for Political and Economic Planning, *Report on the British Health Services* (London: PEP, 1937) and early drafts, notes and comments on the report available in the papers of PEP at the London School of Economics and Political Science.

Secondary sources include: for broadcasting, the four volumes of Asa Briggs, *The History of Broadcasting in the United Kingdom* (London: Oxford University Press, 1961-1979); for film, Rachel Lowe, *The History of British Film, 1929-1939*, 2 vols. (London: George Allen and Unwin, 1979), and Roy Armes, *A Critical History of British Cinema* (London: Secker and Warburg, 1978). The most substantial source on the hospitals and health policy in the thirties is still Brian Abel-Smith, *The Hospitals*. Charles Webster, "Healthy or Hungry Thirties," *History Workshop Journal*, Spring 1982, 5: 10-129, takes a very different perspective; Honigsbaum, *The Division*, details what medical associations did during the thirties. Arthur Marwick, "The Labour Party and the Welfare State in Britain, 1900-48," *American Historical Review*, December 1967, 73: 380-403, and "Middle Opinion in the Thirties: Planning, Progress and Political Agreement," *English Historical Review*, April 1964, 79: 289-298, make substantial contributions. Bentley B. Gilbert, *British Social Policy, 1914-1939*, is still the dominant interpretive study. Paul Adams, *Health of the State* (New York: Praeger, 1982), is a useful comparative study of Britain and the United States in the period, particularly on issues pertaining to public rather than personal health services. His earlier dissertation, cited in the notes, is a more substantial work. The principal secondary sources for the background of PEP are Webster, "Healthy or Hungry Thirties," and Marwick, "Middle Opinion." For Peckham, see Jane Lewis and Barbara Brookes, "The Peckham Health Center, 'PEP' and the Concept of General Practice During the 1930's and 1940's," *Medical History*, 1983, 27: 151-161.

V. Acrimony and Realignment:
The United States, 1932-1940

I studied the perception of medical care in the arts and the media by sampling newspapers, magazines, plays, and novels. An assistant or I examined every article with a title pertaining to medicine or health listed in the *Reader's Guide to Periodical Literature* for the first half of the century. We assessed medical coverage in *Life* by examining every issue published during the magazine's first decade. Generalizations about photography in the 1930s are grounded in the study of images collected by the Center for the Study of Photographic Images of Medicine and Health Care at Stony Brook and, as they relate to the New Deal, the extensive collection of photographs taken for the Farm Security Administration that are in the Manuscript Division of the Library of Congress. See the *Illustrated Catalogue of the Slide Archive of Historical Medical Photographs at Stony Brook* (Westport: Greenwood Press, 1984).

Data about the growth of the health sector of the American economy during the 1930s were derived by compiling statistics published by the federal government and by the American Medical Association. Government sources include: United States Department of Commerce, *National Income and Product of the United States* (Washington, D.C.: USGPO, 1951); and William Weinfeld, *Income of Physicians, 1929-1949* (Washington, D.C.: United States Office of Business Economics, 1950). The data about the growth of hospitals and their increasing utilization were derived by aggregating and analyzing the information that was published annually between 1906 and 1953 by the Council on Medical Education and Hospitals of the American Medical Association.

My analysis of popular culture owes a considerable debt to recent secondary sources in cultural and intellectual history. Notable examples are: Warren I. Sussman, "The Thirties," in Stanley Coben, ed., *The Development of an American Culture* (Englewood Cliffs: Prentice Hall, 1970); Robert Sklar, *Movie Made America: A Social History of the Movies* (New York: Random House, 1975); Malcolm Goldstein, *The Political Stage: American Drama and Theater of the Great Depression* (New York: Oxford University Press, 1974); Raymond William Stedman, *The Serials* (Norman: University of Oklahoma Press, 1971); and James Harvey Young, *The Medical Messiahs* (Princeton: Princeton University Press, 1967).

There are no adequate secondary sources on the modern growth of the hospital industry. Many of the best primary sources and industry polemics, however, contain useful analyses of retrospective data. |Stevens's *American Medicine* remains' an important analysis.

Primary sources on lay reformers include: the vast manuscript and pamphlet collection in the Michael M. Davis Papers; an extensive periodical literature, listed in both *Index Medicus* and the *Reader's Guide to Periodical Literature*; publications of the Committee on Economic Security and the Interdepartmental Committee to Coordinate Health and Welfare Activities; and numerous volumes of congressional hearings. The few pertinent memoirs are cited in the notes.

Doctors, like reformers, published extensively: their articles are accessible through *Index Medicus* and the *Reader's Guide*. My assistant arrayed the titles of every possibly pertinent article in each of these indices between 1900 and 1950. I then selected articles to read on the basis of rough inductive typologies. In addition, there is an extensive literature of histories of state and county medical societies. Most of these books are compilations of primary sources from local societies' manuscript collections. Medical intellectuals, like lay reformers, were forthright about their own opinions; published works by Hugh Cabot and Ernest Boas are particularly revealing. Many of these doctors had extensive correspondence with Michael Davis, which is preserved in his Papers.

There are no definitive secondary studies of either lay or medical reformers in this period. A preliminary analysis of the use of economic analysis by reformers is in D. M. Fox, *Economists and Health Care*. Helpful studies include: Arthur E. Viseltear, "C. E.-A Winslow: His Era and His Contributions to Medical Care," in Charles E. Rosenberg, ed., *Healing and History* (New York: Science History Publications, 1979), and "The California Medical-Economic Survey: Paul A. Dodd vs. the California Medical Association," *Bulletin of the History of Medicine*, March-April 1970, 44: 141-153; and Richard V. Kasius, ed., *The Challenge of Facts: Selected Public Health Papers of Edgard Sydenstriker* (New York: Prodist, 1974). Daniel Hirshfield, *The Lost Reform* (Cambridge: Harvard University Press, 1970), is the best secondary source for both the development of the medical care provisions of the Social Security Act and the Interdepartmental Committee. A useful study of social security, from a general social policy perspective, is Theron F. Schlaback, *Edwin E. Witte: Cautious Reformer* (Madison: State Historical Society of Wisconsin, 1969). The Mary E. Switzer papers at the Schlesinger Library, Radcliffe College, provide an insider's view of politics and policy in the Public Health Service between the mid-1930s and the early 1950s.

The AMA has been as inadequately served by historians as have its enemies. James G. Burrow, *AMA: Voice of American Medicine* (Baltimore: Johns Hopkins University Press, 1963), is detailed, but biased toward reformers. The best description and most compelling interpretation of AMA political activity in the 1930s remains Oliver Garceau, *The Political Life of the American Medical Association* (Cambridge: Harvard University Press, 1941).

VI. THE SECOND WORLD WAR AND HEALTH POLICY: BRITAIN, 1939-1945

Primary sources include: Ministry of Health documents; Cabinet Papers, and documents bearing on the Beveridge Report in the Public Record Office; John Pater, *The Making of the National Health Service* (London: King Edward's Fund, 1982); the British Hospitals Contributory Schemes Papers; the papers in the BMA Registry; the papers of the Society of Medical Officers of Health; Hansard, *Parliamentary Debates*; miscellaneous publications of the Nuffield Provincial Hospitals Trust and King Edward's Hospital Fund for London; and a voluminous pamphlet and periodical literature, much of it conveniently collected in the papers of the Ministry of Health and of the British Hospitals Contributory Schemes.

Secondary sources include: on wartime medical care, C. L. Dunn, *The Emergency Medical Services*, 2 vols. (London: HMSO, 1952), and Richard M. Titmuss, *Problems of Social Policy* (London: HMSO and Longman's Green, 1950); on Beveridge, José Harris, *William Beveridge* (Oxford: Clarendon Press, 1977); on doctors, F. Honigsbaum, *The Division*; on planning for a National Health Service, Harry Eckstein, *The English Health Service* (Cambridge: Harvard University Press, 1958), A. J. Willocks, *The Creation of the National Health Service* (London: Routledge and Kegan Paul, 1967), and Brian Watkin, *The National Health Service: The First Phase* (London: George Allen and Unwin, 1978); on general social policy, Paul Addison, *The Road to 1945* (London: Jonathon Cape, 1975), and J. M. Lee, *The Churchill Coalition* (London: Batsford Academic and Educational, 1980).

VII. THE SECOND WORLD WAR AND HEALTH POLICY: THE UNITED STATES, 1941-1946

Primary sources include: for medicine and culture, an extensive periodical literature, augmented in these years by propaganda for the development of a consensus on policy among interest groups; the reports and supporting documents published during the latter years of the war by the American Hospital Association and the New York Academy of Medicine; for the development of a coalition, the articles and speeches of George Bugbee and Dr. Vane Hoge, which are cited in the notes; and for the federal government, the extensive publications of the United States Public Health Service and the testimony taken by congressional committees, notably by Senator Claude Pepper's Committee on Wartime Health and Education; for the Hill-Burton Act, principal primary sources are the House and Senate Hearings and floor debates, which are cited in the notes, the pamphlet material that was collected by Michael Davis and deposited with his papers and Box 92, General Classified Records, USPHS, Surgeon General's Files, National Archives of the United States.

The outstanding secondary source for the development of public policy for medical care during the war is Monte M. Poen, *Harry S. Truman Versus the Medical Lobby*. Hirshfield, *The Lost Reform*, is helpful. A recent article on the development of the Hill-Burton Act is Dan Feshbach, "What's Inside the Black Box . . . ," *International Journal of Health Services*, no. 2, 1979: 313-339. Marion Ashley Buck, "An American Experiment: Cooperation for Health: A Study of the Hill-Burton Hospital Construction Act of 1946" (unpublished dissertation, Harvard University, 1953), is a useful compilation of data. On congressional politics: Stephen K. Bailey, *Congress Makes a Law* (New York: Columbia University Press, 1950) and James T. Patterson, *Mr. Republican* (Boston: Houghton Mifflin Co., 1972).

VIII. ESTABLISHING THE NATIONAL HEALTH SERVICE: BRITAIN, 1946-1951

Principal primary sources include: Ministry of Health and Cabinet Papers; Papers of the British Hospitals Contributory Schemes Association; John Pater, *The Making of the National Health Service*; Hansard; the pamphlet and periodical literature and the reports and regulations issued by the Ministry of Health in the early years of the NHS. For the period to early 1954, some ministry and Cabinet papers in the Public Record Office were available to me, but many pertinent files remain closed because they contain material that bears on later events. Hansard and reports of Parliamentary Committees were especially useful in the absence of archival material.

The most important secondary source for the history of the NHS is Rudolf Klein, *The Politics of the National Health Service* (London:

Longman, 1983). Klein's book is valuable for the war years as well as for the period covered in this and subsequent chapters. Other important secondary sources on politics include Michael Foot, *Aneurin Bevan: A Biography*, 2 vols. (New York: Atheneum, 1963, 1974); Neville M. Goodman, *Wilson Jameson: Architect of National Health* (London: George Allen and Unwin, 1970); A.C.H. Smith, *Paper Voices: The Popular Press and Social Change, 1935-65* (London: Chatto and Windus, 1975); Harry Eckstein, *Pressure Group Politics: The Case of the British Medical Association* (London: George Allen and Unwin, 1960), compares the BMA and the AMA. General books include, Roger Eatwell, *The 1945-51 Labour Governments* (London: B. T. Batsford Ltd., 1979). Kenneth Morgan, *Labour in Power, 1945-51* (Oxford: Clarendon Press, 1984), which argues a thesis at variance with mine; and Henry Pelling, *The Labour Governments, 1945-51* (New York: St. Martin's Press, 1984). Secondary sources on NHS administration include James Stirling Ross, *The National Health Service in Great Britain*; J. A. Griffith, *Central Departments and Local Authorities* (London: George Allen and Unwin, 1966), and R.G.S. Brown, *Reorganizing the National Health Service: a Case Study in Administrative Change* (Oxford: Basil Blackwell, 1979).

IX. A POLICY FOR GROWTH:
THE UNITED STATES, 1946-1953

The most useful source for opinion about health policy is the periodical and monographic literature. There are a number of useful contemporary books about doctors, including: Morris Fishbein, *An Autobiography* (New York: Doubleday, 1969); James Howard Means, *Doctors, People and Government* (Boston: Little, Brown, 1953); and, most important, Ernest Dichter, *A Psychological Study of the Doctor-Patient Relationship* (Sacramento: California Medical Association, 1950). Senator Paul Douglas's autobiography, *In the Fullness of Time* (New York: Harcourt Brace Jovanovich, 1972) provides compelling data about liberals' attitudes toward health policy and the perception of the AMA among professional politicians. Public reports, which were usually generated in order to press for new policy, include: The President's Scientific Research Board, *The Nation's Research: Science and Public Policy; A Report to the President*, vol. 5 (Washington, D.C.: USGPO, 1947); National Health Assembly, *America's Health* (New York: Harper and Brothers, 1949); Oscar Ewing, *The Nation's Health: A Report to the President* (Washington, D.C.: U.S. Federal Security Agency, 1948); and President's Commission on the

Health Needs of the Nation, *Building America's Health*, 4 vols. (Washington, D.C.: USGPO, 1952). Extensive manuscript records of the commission's deliberations are in the Harry S. Truman Library, Independence, Missouri.

Secondary and primary sources are difficult to separate for events that are so recent. I label as secondary studies those in which journalists or scholars tried to be detached rather than explicitly polemic. Such studies include: for perceptions of medical care, Jacob J. Feldman, *The Dissemination of Health Information* (Chicago: Aldine, 1966), and Monroe Lerner and Odin W. Anderson, *Health Progress in the United States, 1900-1960* (Chicago: University of Chicago Press, 1963); for the growth of constituencies to increase the supply of medical care, facilities and research, James Harvey Young, *The Medical Messiahs*, Stephen Strickland, *Politics, Science, and Dread Disease*, and E. L. Koos, *The Health of Regionville* (New York: Hafner, 1967 [1954]); for doctors' political behavior, James G. Burrow, *AMA: Voice of American Medicine*, and Richard Harris, *A Sacred Trust* (New York: New American Library, 1966); on the Truman Administration, Monte Poen, *Harry S. Truman*, the essays and citations in Richard Kirkendall, ed., *The Truman Period as a Research Field: A Reappraisal* (Columbia: University of Missouri Press, 1974); Alonzo L. Hamby, *Beyond the New Deal: Harry S. Truman and American Liberalism* (New York: Columbia University Press, 1973), and a number of monographs that are cited in the notes. A useful study, with an interpretation that differs markedly from mine, is Odin W. Anderson, *The Uneasy Equilibrium: Private and Public Financing of Health Services in the United States, 1875-1965* (New Haven: College and University Press, 1968). The only study of the history of the Public Health Service is Bess Furman, *A Profile of the United States Public Health Service* (Washington, D.C.: USGPO, 1973). Stevens, *American Medicine*, remains an indispensable book for the history of policy and health institutions. A useful recent synthesis is Odin W. Anderson, *Health Services in the United States: A Growth Enterprise Since 1875* (Ann Arbor: Health Administration Press, 1985).

X. The Priorities of the National Health Service: Britain, 1951-1962

Because of the rule limiting access to papers in the Public Record Office for thirty years, there are few manuscript sources on policy formation since 1954. Charles Webster, Walter Holland, and Rudolf Klein helped me to understand published sources. The Society of Medical

Officers of Health Papers were useful. Parliamentary Debates were helpful, as was the information about priorities obtained by reading subject headings in the annual indices to them. An indispensable published source is Brian Abel-Smith and Richard Titmuss, *The Cost of the National Health Service* (Cambridge: Cambridge University Press, 1956) A major source for context was a report to the Rockefeller Foundation by Osler L. Peterson, its official observer in Britain during the formative years of the NHS, *A Study of the National Health Service of Great Britain* (New York: the Rockefeller Foundation, 1951, processed). An important source is Department of Health and Social Security, *Review of Health Capital: A Discussion Document on the Role of Capital in the Provision of Health Services* (London: DHSS, October 1979), which contains magnificent tables and a cogent historical analysis by Jonathan Tross of the ministry.

Much of the material on both Britain and the United States since the 1950s has been culled from my work, over a period of years, in health services research. Scholars in this field ask different questions from historians. As the field has matured, its data and generalizations have provided a solid basis for historical work. An exemplary work in the British literature of health sciences research is John R. Butler, J. M. Bevan, R. C. Taylor, *Family Doctors and Public Policy: A Study of Manpower Distribution* (London: Routledge and Kegan Paul, 1973). More important, the numerous articles and recent book by Rudolf Klein are indispensable for comprehending the history of the NHS. The many volumes published by the Nuffield Trust, under the editorship of Gordon McLachlan, contain essays of great importance for the history of the NHS. For many years this series of volumes was titled *Problems and Progress in Medical Care* (London: Oxford University Press). A useful monograph, which is, however, deficient in its use of historical methodology is David E. Allen, *Hospital Planning: The Development of the 1962 Hospital Plan* (London: Pitman Medical 1979). A helpful source for British demography is J. N. Morris, *Uses of Epidemiology*, 3rd edition (Edinburgh and London: Churchill Livingstone, 1975).

Samuel H. Beer, *Modern British Politics* (London: Faber and Faber, 1965), was indispensable background for much of this book but is particularly important for the analysis in this chapter because Beer uses historical data to explain British politics in the 1950s and 1960s and to compare them with contemporary institutions and events in the United States. Another useful source for comparative politics is Arnold J. Heidenheimer, "The Politics of Public Education, Health and Welfare in the USA and Western Europe: How Growth and Re-

form Potentials Have Differed," *British Journal of Political Science,*
July 1973, 3: 315-340.

XI. A Triumphant Coalition:
The United States, 1953-1965

Primary sources include: numerous public reports, particularly by
staff and consultants to the Public Health Service and to the Secretary of Health, Education and Welfare and by staff members of
congressional committees; congressional hearings and debates; and
the general and professional periodical literature. Vernon W. Lippard and Elizabeth F. Purcell, eds., *Case Histories of Ten New Medical
Schools* (New York: Josiah Macy, Jr., Foundation, 1972) collects
eyewitness accounts of the development of local coalitions pressing
to increase the supply of medical services. The dominant monograph in the field is Rosemary Stevens, *American Medicine.* Studies
of the labor movement include John T. Dunlop and Walter Galenson, eds., *Labor in the Twentieth Century* (New York: Academic Press,
1978); Duncan M. MacIntyre, *Voluntary Health Insurance and Rate
Making* (Ithaca: Cornell University Press, 1962); Raymond Munts,
Bargaining for Health: Labor Unions, Health Insurance and Medical Care
(Madison: University of Wisconsin Press, 1967); and J. F. Follman,
Medical Care and Health Insurance (Homewood: Richard D. Irwin,
1963). Odin Anderson, *Uneasy Equilibrium* is a useful narrative history of events in the period. Notable accounts of the political history
of Medicare are Theodore R. Marmor, *The Politics of Medicare* (Chi-
cago: Aldine, 1970); Max J. Skidmore, *Medicare and the American
Rhetoric of Reconciliation* (Montgomery: University of Alabama Press,
1970); and Howard Berliner, "The Origins of Health Insurance for
the Aged," *International Journal of Health Services,* Summer 1973, 3:
465-474. Monographs on medical care policy in the 1960s include
Martha Derthick, *Policymaking for Social Security* (Washington:
Brookings Institution, 1979); David E. Price, *Who Makes the Laws?
Creativity and Power in Senate Committees* (Cambridge: Schenkman
Publishing Co., 1972); and Judith M. Feder, *Medicare: The Politics of
Federal Hospital Insurance* (Lexington: D. C. Heath and Co., 1977),
which describes the implementation of medicare and documents
how members of the groups in the dominant coalition accommo-
dated to each other.

INDEX

Abel-Smith, Brian, 175-176, 179, 185
Addison, Christopher, 8, 38, 47; appoints consultative council, 28-30; creation of Ministry of Health, 22-26, 34
Altmeyer, Arthur, 91, 123, 152-153
American Association for Labor Legislation, 5, 10-11, 13, 14, 89
American College of Physicians, 84
American College of Surgeons, 84
American Economic Association, 153
American Federation of Labor, 12, 120. *See also* organized labor
American Foundation, *American Medicine: Expert Testimony Out of Court*, 87-88
American Hospital Association, advocates changes in health policy, 117; alliance with U.S. Public Health Service, 120, 120n; Commission on Hospital Care, 118-119, 121-122, 131; endorses hierarchical regionalism, 118; policy agenda changes, 198; supports federal hospital construction, 92-93; supports Hill-Burton Act, 124
American Medical Association, adjusts to diversity of medical practice, 196-197, 197n; attacks CCMC majority report, 50-51; Bureau of Medical Economics, 83; Committee on Postwar Service, 122; concern of members over specialization, 153-156; continued resistance to prepaid group practice, 197n; Council on Medical Education and Hospitals, 41, 167, 192; influence on physicians, 84-85; and perceived shortage of doctors, 192-194, 192n; political influence of, 156-158, 156n, 157n, 158n; position on national health insurance, 12, 39, 86; position on National Health Program, 90, 92, 92n, 127; and reform of medical education, 39, 41, 45; resistance to hierarchical regionalism, 42-43; resistance to Medicare, 203-205, 203n, 204n; Section on General Practice, 154
Annis, Edward, 204, 205
Appel, James, 204, 205
Association of American Medical Colleges, 167, 198
Association of Municipal Corporations, 98-99
Astor, Waldorf, 24
Attlee, Clement, 113; compromise on National Health Service, 145-148; speech on National Health Service, 140-141

Bevan, Aneurin, accepts physician autonomy, 143n, 148; advocates central role for hospitals, 179; compared to Lister Hill, 138; and cost of National Health Service, 174; National Health Service's financial crisis, 144-146; position on National Health Service's financial crisis, 144-146; proposals for a national health service, 179n; sets Sir Cyril Jones' findings aside, 148n; speech on National Health Service Bill, 137-138; supports nationalizing hospitals, 133-135, 134n, 137n
Beveridge, Sir William, 105n, 114, 144, 175, 177n, 211; and Beveridge Report, 104-106, 135; consensus on, within medical profession, 106n
Bevin, Ernest, 113
Biggs, Hermann N., 37, 42
Bingham Associates Fund, 165
Boas, Ernest, 87
Brackenbury, Sir Henry, 57, 58
Brend, William, 9-10, 32
British Hospital Association, 7, 133; appoints committee to implement Sankey Report, 59; establishes Voluntary Hospital Commission, 58; supports a national health service, 96, 108n, 110, 112, 137, 140; supports regional hierarchies, 58

227